How to Write a Paper

Third edition

How to Write a Paper

Third edition

Edited by

George M Hall

*Department of Anaesthesia and Intensive Care Medicine,
St George's Hospital Medical School, London*

© BMJ Publishing Group 2003

BMJ Books is an imprint of the BMJ Publishing Group

First published in 1994
by the BMJ Publishing Group, BMA House, Tavistock Square,
London WC1H 9JR

First edition 1994
Reprinted 1994, 1995, 1996, 1997, 1998
Second edition 1998
Reprinted 1999
Reprinted 2000
Reprinted 2002
Third edition 2003
6   2007

British Library Cataloguing in Publication Data

A catalogue record for this book is available from the British Library

ISBN 978-0-7279-1728-7

Cover design by Dellaway

Typeset by SIVA Math Setters, Chennai, India
Printed and bound in Spain by GraphyCems, Navarra

Contents

Contributors

Robert N Allan
Consultant Gastroenterologist, Queen Elizabeth Hospital, Birmingham, UK

Craig Bingham
Manager, Communications Development, Medical Journal of Australia, Pyrmont, Australia

Margaret Cooter
Managing Technical Editor, BMJ Publishing Group, London, UK

Natalie Davies
Project Manager, BMJ Publishing Group, London, UK

Michael Doherty
Professor of Rheumatology, Academic Rheumatology, University of Nottingham Medical School, City Hospital, Nottingham, UK

Gordon B Drummond
University Department of Anaesthesia, Critical Care, and Pain Medicine, Edinburgh, UK

Michael JG Farthing
Executive Dean, Faculty of Medicine, University of Glasgow, Glasgow, UK

Ian Forgacs
Consultant Physician, Department of Gastroenterology, King's College Hospital, London, UK

George M Hall
Department of Anaesthesia and Intensive Care Medicine, St George's Hospital Medical School, London, UK

Richard Horton
Editor, *Lancet,* London, UK

Simon Howell
Academic Unit of Anaesthesia, Leeds General Infirmary, Leeds, UK

Domhnall MacAuley
Department of Epidemiology and Public Health, The Queen's University of Belfast, Belfast and Associate Editor, *BMJ*, London, UK

Harvey Marcovitch
Syndications Editor, BMJ Journals, London, UK

Fiona Moss
Associate Dean, London Deanery, London Department of Postgraduate Medical and Dental Education, and Editor, *Quality and Safety in Health Care*, London, UK

Hans-Joachim Priebe
Professor of Anaesthesia, Department of Anaesthesia, University Hospital Freiburg, Freiburg, Germany

G Smith
Professor of Anaesthesia, Leicester Warwick Medical School, Leicester, UK

Richard Smith
Editor, *BMJ*, London, UK

Leo van de Putte
Professor of Rheumatology, University Hospital Nijmegen, Department of Rheumatology, Nijmegen, Netherlands

JAW Wildsmith
University Department of Anaesthesia, Ninewells Hospital and Medical School, Dundee, UK

Alex Williamson
Publishing Director, BMJ Journals and Books, London, UK

Preface to third edition

The unexpected success of the first and second editions of this short book and the rapid progress in certain areas of publishing have necessitated a third edition. The original intention was that it would appeal primarily to authors for whom English was not their first language. Sales in the United Kingdom, however, show that it has met a local need. For the third edition, it is a pleasure to welcome Craig Bingham, Margaret Cooter, Natalie Davies, Simon Howell, Domhnall MacAuley, Harvey Marcovitch, Fiona Moss, Hans-Joachim Priebe, and Leo van de Putte as new contributors. An additional chapter, "Electronic submissions," has been added.

I am grateful to all authors for revising their chapters and, in particular, to Robert Allan, Michael Doherty, Gordon Drummond, Graham Smith, Richard Smith, Tony Wildsmith, and Alex Williamson for contributing to all three editions.

George M Hall

1: Structure of a scientific paper

GEORGE M HALL

The research you have conducted is obviously of vital importance and must be read by the widest possible audience. It probably is safer to insult a colleague's spouse, family, and driving than the quality of his or her research. Fortunately, so many medical journals now exist that your chances of not having the work published somewhere are small. Nevertheless, the paper must be constructed in the approved manner and presented to the highest possible standards. Editors and assessors without doubt will look adversely on scruffy manuscripts – regardless of the quality of the science. All manuscripts are constructed in a similar manner, although some notable exceptions exist, like the format used by *Nature*. Such exceptions are unlikely to trouble you in the early stages of your research career.

The object of publishing a scientific paper is to provide a document that contains sufficient information to enable readers to:

- assess the observations you made
- repeat the experiment if they wish
- determine whether the conclusions drawn are justified by the data.

The basic structure of a paper is summarised by the acronym IMRAD, which stands for:

Introduction   (What question was asked?)
Methods   (How was it studied?)
Results   (What was found?)
And
Discussion   (What do the findings mean?)

The next four chapters of this book each deal with a specific section of a paper, so the sections will be described only in outline in this chapter.

Introduction

The introduction should be brief and must state clearly the question that you tried to answer in the study. To lead the reader to this point, it is necessary to review the relevant literature briefly.

Many junior authors find it difficult to write the introduction. The most common problem is the inability to state clearly what question was asked. This should not be a problem if the study was planned correctly – it is too late to rectify basic errors when attempting to write the paper. Nevertheless, some studies seem to develop a life of their own, and the original objectives can easily be forgotten. I find it useful to ask collaborators from time to time what question we hope to answer. If I do not receive a short clear sentence as an answer, then alarm bells ring.

The introduction must not include a review of the literature. Only cite those references that are essential to justify your proposed study. Three citations from different groups usually are enough to convince most assessors that some fact is "well known" or "well recognised," particularly if the studies are from different countries. Many research groups write the introduction to a paper before the work is started, but you must never ignore pertinent literature published while the study is in progress.

An example introduction might be:

It is well known that middle-aged male runners have diffuse brain damage,[1–3] but whether this is present before they begin running or arises as a result of repeated cerebral contusions during exercise has not been established. In the present study, we examined cerebral function in a group of sedentary middle-aged men before and after a six month exercise programme. Cerebral function was assessed by ...

Methods

This important part of the manuscript increasingly is neglected, and yet the methods section is the most common cause of absolute rejection of a paper. If the methods used to try to answer the question were inappropriate or flawed, then there is no salvation for the work. Chapter 3 contains useful advice about the design of the study and precision of measurement that should be considered when the work is planned – not after the work has been completed.

The main purposes of the methods section are to describe, and sometimes defend, the experimental design and to provide enough detail that a competent worker could repeat the study. The latter is particularly important when you are deciding how much to include in the text. If standard methods of measurement are used, appropriate references are all that is required. In many instances, "modifications" of published methods are used, and it is these that cause difficulties for other workers. To ensure reproducible data, authors should:

- give complete details of any new methods used
- give the precision of the measurements undertaken
- sensibly use statistical analysis.

The use of statistics is not covered in this book. Input from a statistician should be sought at the planning stage of any study. Statisticians invariably are helpful, and they have contributed greatly to improving both the design and analysis of clinical investigations. They cannot be expected, however, to resurrect a badly designed study.

Results

The results section of a paper has two key features: there should be an overall description of the major findings of the study; and the data should be presented clearly and concisely.

You do not need to present every scrap of data that you have collected. A great temptation is to give all the results, particularly if they were difficult to obtain, but this section should contain only relevant, representative data. The statistical analysis of the results must be appropriate. The easy availability of statistical software packages has not encouraged young research workers to understand the principles involved. An assessor is only able to estimate the validity of the statistical tests used, so if your analysis is complicated or unusual, expect your paper to undergo appraisal by a statistician.

You must strive for clarity in the results section by avoiding unnecessary repetition of data in the text, figures, and tables. It is worthwhile stating briefly what you did *not* find, as this may stop other workers in the area undertaking unnecessary studies.

Discussion

The initial draft of the discussion is almost invariably too long. It is difficult not to write a long and detailed analysis of the literature that you know so well. A rough guide to the length of this section, however, is that it should not be more than one third of the total length of the manuscript (Introduction + Methods + Results + Discussion). Ample scope often remains for further pruning.

Many beginners find this section of the paper difficult. It is possible to compose an adequate discussion around the points given in Box 1.1.

Common errors include repetition of data already given in the results section, a belief that the methods were beyond criticism, and preferential citing of previous work to suit the conclusions. Good assessors will seize upon such mistakes, so do not even contemplate trying to deceive them.

Although IMRAD describes the basic structure of a paper, other parts of a manuscript are important. The title, summary (or abstract), and list of authors are described in Chapter 6. It is salutary to remember that many people will read the title of the paper and some will read the summary, but very few will read the complete text. The title and summary of the paper are

---

Box 1.1 Writing the discussion

- Summarise the major findings
- Discuss possible problems with the methods used
- Compare your results with previous work
- Discuss the clinical and scientific (if any) implications of your findings
- Suggest further work
- Produce a succinct conclusion

of great importance for indexing and abstracting purposes, as well as enticing readers to peruse the complete text. The use of appropriate references for a paper is described in Chapter 7; this section often is full of mistakes. A golden rule is to list only relevant, published references and to present them in a manner that is appropriate for the particular journal to which the article is being submitted. The citation of large numbers of references is an indicator of insecurity – not of scholarship. An authoritative author knows the important references that are appropriate to the study.

Before you start the first draft of the manuscript, carefully read the "Instructions to authors" that every journal publishes, and prepare your paper accordingly. Some journals give detailed instructions, often annually, and these can be a valuable way of learning some of the basic rules. A grave mistake is to submit a paper to one journal in the style of another; this suggests that it has recently been rejected. At all stages of preparation of the paper, go back and check with the instructions to authors to make sure that your manuscript conforms. It seems very obvious, but if you wish to publish in the *European Annals of Andrology*, do not write your paper to conform with the *Swedish Journal of Androgen Research*. Read and re-read the instructions to authors.

Variations on the IMRAD system are sometimes necessary in specialised circumstances, such as a letter to the editor (Chapter 9), an abstract for presentation at a scientific meeting (Chapter 10), or a case report (Chapter 11). Nevertheless, a fundamental structure is the basis of all scientific papers.

2: Introductions

RICHARD SMITH

Introductions should be short and arresting, and they should tell the reader why you have undertaken the study. This first sentence tells you almost everything I have to say and you could stop here. If you were reading a newspaper, you probably would – and that is why a journalist writing a news story will try to give the essence of their story in the first line. An alternative technique used by journalists and authors is to begin with a sentence so arresting that the reader will be hooked and is likely to stay for the whole piece.

I may mislead by beginning with these journalistic devices, but I want to return to them: scientific writing can borrow usefully from journalism. Let me begin, however, with writing introductions for scientific papers.

Before you begin, answer the basic questions

Before you sit down to write an introduction, you must have answered the basic questions that apply to any piece of writing:

- What do I have to say?
- Is it worth saying?
- What is the right format for the message?
- What is the audience for the message?
- What is the right journal for the message?

If you are unclear about the answers to these questions, your piece of writing – no matter whether it's a news story, a poem, or a scientific paper – is unlikely to succeed. As editor of the *BMJ*, every day I see papers in which the authors have not answered these questions. Authors often are not clear about what they want to say; they start with some sort of idea and hope that the reader will have the wit to sort out what's important. The reader will not bother. Authors also regularly choose the wrong format – a scientific paper rather than a descriptive essay, or a long paper rather than a short one. Not being clear about the audience is probably the most common error, and specialists regularly write for generalists in a way that is entirely inaccessible.

Another basic rule is to read the "Instructions to authors" of the journal you are writing for (or "Advice to contributors," as politically correct journals such as the *BMJ* now call them). Too few authors do this, but there is little point in writing a 400 word introduction when the journal has a limit for the whole article of 600 words.

Tell readers why you have undertaken the study

The main job of the introduction is to tell readers why you have undertaken the study. You will have little difficulty if you set out to answer a question that really interested you. But, if your main reason for undertaking the study was to have something to add to your curriculum vitae, it will show. The best questions may arise directly from clinical practice, and, if that is the case, the introduction should say so:

> A patient was anaesthetised for an operation to repair his hernia and asked whether the fact that he used Ecstasy four nights a week would cause problems. We were unable to find an answer in published medical reports, and so we designed a study to answer the question.

Or:

> Because of pressure to reduce night work for junior doctors we wondered if it would be safe to delay operating on patients with appendicitis until the morning after they were admitted.

If your audience is interested in the answer to these questions, they may well be tempted to read the paper, and, if you have defined your audience and selected the right journal, they should be interested.

More often, you will be building on scientific work already published. It then is essential to make clear how your work adds importantly to what has gone before.

Clarify what your work adds

Editors will not want to publish – and readers will not want to read – studies that simply repeat what has been done several times before. Indeed, you should not be undertaking a study or writing a paper unless you are confident that it adds importantly to what has gone before. The introduction should not read:

Several studies have shown that regular Ecstasy use creates anaesthetic difficulties,[1–7] and several others have shown that it does not.[8–14] We report two further patients, one of whom experienced problems and one of whom did not, and we review the literature.

It rather should read something like:

Two previous studies have reported that regular Ecstasy use may give rise to respiratory problems during anaesthesia. These studies were small and uncontrolled, used only crude measurements of respiratory function, and did not follow up the patients. We report a larger, controlled study, with detailed measurements of respiratory function and two year follow up.

Usually, it is not so easy to make clear how your study is better than previous studies, and this is where you might be tempted to give a detailed critique of everything that has ever gone before. You will be particularly tempted to do this because, if you are serious about your study, you will have spent hours in the library detecting and reading all the relevant literature. The very best introductions include a systematic review of all the work that has gone before and a demonstration that new work is needed.

The move towards systematic reviews is one of the most important developments in science and scientific writing in the past 20 years.[1] We now understand that most reviews are highly selective in the evidence they adduce and that they often are wrong in the conclusions they reach.[2] When an author undertakes a systematic review, they pose a clear question, gather all relevant information (published in whatever language or unpublished), discard the scientifically weak material, synthesise the remaining information, and then draw a conclusion.

To undertake such a review is clearly a major task, but this ideally is what you should do before you begin a new study.

You then should undertake the study only if the question cannot be answered and if your study will contribute importantly towards producing an answer. You should include a brief account of the review in the introduction. Readers will then fully understand how your study fits with what has gone before and why it is important.

"In 2003 you should not worry that you cannot reach this high standard because the number of medical papers that have ever done so could probably be numbered on the fingers of one hand." I wrote the same sentence in the first edition of this book but with the year as 1994 and in the second edition with the year as 1998. I then wrote in the first edition: "But by the end of the millennium brief accounts of such reviews will, I hope, be routine in introductions." I was – as always – wildly overoptimistic. Summaries of systematic reviews are still far from routine in introductions in scientific papers. Indeed, a paper presented at the Third International Congress on Peer Review in September 1997 showed that many randomised controlled trials published in the world's five major general medical journals failed to mention trials previously done on the same subject.

This means that authors routinely are flouting the Helsinki Declaration on research involving human subjects. The declaration states that such research should be based on a thorough knowledge of the scientific literature.[3] Repetition of research that has been done satisfactorily already is poor practice. As the CONSORT statement on good practice in reporting clinical trials says: "Some clinical trials have been shown to have been unnecessary, because the question they addressed had been or could have been answered by a systematic review of the existing literature."[4,5]

In 2003, my advice on systematically reviewing previous reports remains a counsel of perfection, but it is still good advice. Perhaps you can be somebody who moves scientific papers forward, rather than somebody who just reaches the minimum standard for publication.

Another important and relevant advance since the first edition is that almost all scientific journals now have websites and publish synergistically on paper and on the web.[6,7] This at last opens up the possibility of being able to satisfy simultaneously the needs of the reader–researcher, who wants lots of detail and data, and the needs of the reader–practitioner, who wants a straightforward message. The *BMJ*, for example, has introduced a system it calls ELPS (electronic long, paper short).[8] In this case, the editors produce the shorter paper, although it is approved by the authors before publication. In the context of introductions, this synergistic publishing might mean that a proper systematic review is published on the web, while the paper version might include a short and simple summary. Usually, however, a full systematic review is probably best dealt with as a separate paper.

Follow the best advice

An important development in medical writing in the past five years has been the appearance of suggested structures for certain kinds of studies. These have appeared because of considerable evidence that many scientific reports do not include important information. Guidelines have been created for randomised controlled trials,[4] systematic reviews,[9] economic evaluations,[10] and, most recently, studies that report on tests of diagnostic methods.[11] More guidelines will follow – for example, on qualitative studies – and many journals, including the *BMJ*, will require authors to conform to these standards and will send back reports that do not conform. Authors thus need to be aware of these guidelines. The requirements for introductions are usually straightforward and not very different from the advice given in this chapter.

Keep it short

You must resist the temptation to impress readers by summarising everything that has gone before. They will be bored – not impressed – and will probably never make it through your study. Your introduction should not read:

Archaeologists have hypothesised that a primitive version of Ecstasy may have been used widely in ancient Egypt. Canisters found in tombs of the pharaohs ... Sociological evidence shows that Ecstasy is most commonly used by males aged 15 to 25 at parties held in aircraft hangars ... The respiratory problems associated with Ecstasy may arise at the alveolar – capillary interface. Aardvark hypothesised in 1926 that problems might arise at this interface because of...

Nor should you write:

Many studies have addressed the problem of Ecstasy and anaesthesia.[1–9]

With such sentences, you say almost nothing useful and you've promptly filled a whole page with references. You should choose references that are apposite, not use references simply to show that you've done a lot of reading.

It may often be difficult to make clear in a few words why your study is superior to previous studies, but you must convince editors and readers that yours is better. Your introduction might read something like:

Anaesthetists cannot be sure whether important complications may arise in patients who regularly use Ecstasy. Several case studies have described such problems.[1–4] Three cohort studies have been published, two of which found a high incidence of respiratory problems in regular Ecstasy users. One of these studies was uncontrolled,[5] and in the other, the patients were matched poorly for age and smoking.[6] The study that did not find any problems included only six regular Ecstasy users, and the chance of an important effect being missed (a type II error) was high.[7] We undertook a study of 50 regular users of Ecstasy, with controls matched for age, smoking status, and alcohol consumption.

A more detailed critique of the other studies should be left for the discussion. Even then, you should not give an exhaustive account of what has gone before but should concentrate on the best studies that are closest to yours. You then also will be able to compare the strengths and weaknesses of your study with the other studies – something that would be wholly out of place in the introduction.

Make sure that you are aware of earlier studies

I've emphasised already the importance of locating earlier studies. Before beginning a study, authors should seek the help of librarians to find any earlier studies. Authors should also make personal contact with people who are experts in the subject and who may know of published studies that library searches do not find, unpublished studies, or studies currently under way. It's also a good idea to find the latest possible review on the subject and search the references and to look at the abstracts of meetings on the subject. We know that library searches often do not find relevant papers that already have been published, that many good studies remain unpublished (perhaps because they reach negative conclusions), and that studies take years to conduct and sometimes years to become published reports.

Editors increasingly want to see evidence that authors have worked hard to make sure they know of studies directly related to theirs. This is particularly important when an editor's first reaction to a paper is "Surely we know this already." We regularly have this experience at the *BMJ* and we then look especially hard to make sure that authors have made an effort at finding what has gone before.

In a systematic review, the search strategy clearly belongs in the methods section, but in an ordinary paper it belongs in the introduction – in as short a form as possible. Thus it might read:

A Medline search with 15 different key phrases, personal contact with five experts in the subject, and a personal search of five recent conferences on closely related subjects produced no previous studies of whether grandmothers suck eggs.

Be sure your readers are convinced of the importance of your question, but don't overdo it

If you have selected the right audience and a good study then you should not have to work hard to convince your readers of the importance of the question you are answering. One common mistake is to start repeating material that is in all the textbooks and that your readers will know. Thus, in a paper on whether vitamin D will prevent osteoporosis, you do not need to explain what osteoporosis and vitamin D are. You might, however, want to give them a sense of the scale of the problem, by including prevalence figures for osteoporosis, data on hospital admissions related to osteoporosis, and figures on the cost of the problem to the nation.

Don't baffle your readers

Although you don't want to patronise and bore your readers by telling them things they already know, you certainly don't want to baffle them by introducing, without explanation, material that is wholly unfamiliar. Nothing turns readers off faster than abbreviations that mean nothing or references to diseases, drugs, reports, places, or whatever that they do not know. This point simply emphasises the importance of knowing your audience.

Give the study's design but not the conclusion

This is a matter of choice, but I ask authors to give a one sentence description of their study at the end of the introduction. The last line might read:

We therefore conducted a double blind randomised study with 10 year follow up to determine whether teetotallers drinking three glasses of whisky a week can reduce their chances of dying of coronary artery disease.

I don't like it, however, when the introduction also gives the final conclusion:

Drinking three glasses of whisky a week does not reduce teetotallers' chances of dying of coronary artery disease.

Other editors may think differently.

Think about using journalistic tricks sparingly

The difficult part of writing is to get the structure right. Spinning sentences is much easier than finding the right structure, and editors can much more easily change sentences than structure. Most pieces of writing that fail do so because the structure is poor; that is why writing scientific articles is comparatively easy – the structure is given to you.

I have assumed in this chapter that you are writing a scientific paper. If you are writing something else, you will have to think much harder about the introduction and about the structure of the whole piece. But even if you are writing a scientific paper, you might make use of devices that journalists use to hook their readers.

Tim Albert, a medical journalist, gives five possible openings in his excellent book on medical journalism:[12]

- telling an arresting story
- describing a scene vividly
- using a strong quotation
- giving some intriguing facts
- making an opinionated and controversial pronouncement.

He gives two examples from the health page of the *Independent*. Mike Hanscomb wrote:

In many respects it is easier and less uncomfortable to have leukaemia than eczema...

This is an intriguing statement, and readers will be interested to read on to see if the author can convince them that his statement contains some truth. Jeremy Laurance began a piece:

This is a story of sex, fear, and money. It is about a new treatment for an embarrassing problem which could prove a money spinner in the new commercial National Health Service...

Sex, fear, and money are emotive to all of us and we may well want to know how a new treatment could make money for the health service rather than costing it money. My favourite beginning occurs in Anthony Burgess's novel *Earthly Powers*. The first sentence reads:

It was the afternoon of my eighty-first birthday, and I was in bed with my catamite when Ali announced that the archbishop had come to see me.

This starts the book so powerfully that it might well carry us right through the next 400 or so pages. (I had to look up "catamite" too. It means "boy kept for homosexual purposes".) To begin a paper in the *British Journal of Anaesthesia* with such a sentence would be to court rejection, ridicule, and disaster, but some of the techniques advocated by Tim Albert could be used. I suggest, however, that you stay away from using opinionated statements and quotations in scientific papers, particularly if they come from Shakespeare, the Bible, or *Alice in Wonderland.*

Conclusion

To write an effective introduction you must know your audience, keep it short, tell readers why you have done the study and explain why it's important, convince readers that it is better than what has gone before, and try as hard as you can to hook them in the first line.

References

1   Chalmers I. Improving the quality and dissemination of reviews of clinical research. In: Lock S, ed. *The future of medical journals.* London: BMJ Books, 1991:127–48.
2   Mulrow CD. The medical review article: state of the science. *Ann Intern Med* 1987;**104**:485–8.
3   World Medical Association. Declaration of Helsinki. Recommendations guiding physicians in biomedical research involving human subjects. *JAMA* 1997;**277**:925–6.
4   Moher D, Schulz KF, Altman DG. The CONSORT statement: revised recommendations for improving the quality of reports of parallel-group randomised trials. *Lancet* 2001;**357**:1191–4.
5   Lau J, Antman EM, Jimenez-Silva J, Kupelnick B, Mosteller F, Chalmers TC. Cumulative meta-analysis of therapeutic trials for myocardial infarction. *N Engl J Med* 1992;**327**:248–54.
6   Bero L, Delamothe T, Dixon A, *et al.* The electronic future: what might an online scientific paper look like in five years' time? *BMJ* 1997;**315**:1692–6.
7   Delamothe T. Is that it? How online articles have changed over the past five years. *BMJ* 2002;**325**:1475–8.
8   Müllner M, Groves T. Making research papers in the BMJ more accessible. *BMJ* 2002;**325**:456.
9   Moher D, Cook DJ, Eastwood S, *et al.* Improving the quality of reports of meta-analyses of randomised controlled trials: the QUOROM statement. Quality of Reporting of Meta-analyses. *Lancet* 1999;**354**:1896–900.
10 Drummond MF, Jefferson TO. Guidelines for authors and peer reviewers of economic submissions to the BMJ. The BMJ Economic Evaluation Working Party. *BMJ* 1996;**313**:275–83.
11 Bossuyt PM, Reitsma B, Bruns DE, *et al.* Towards complete and accurate reporting of studies of diagnostic accuracy: the STARD initiative. *BMJ* 2003;**326**:41–4.
12 Albert T. *Medical journalism: the writer's guide.* Oxford: Radcliffe, 1992.

3: Methods

GORDON B DRUMMOND

The methods section should describe, in logical sequence, how your study was designed and carried out and how you analysed your data. This should be a simple task when the study is complete; however, if you leave writing the methods until this stage, you may only then recognise flaws in the design that you would have detected sooner if you had written this part in as much detail as possible *before* the study started. An experienced colleague could help by looking through this description to find weaknesses. The challenge of setting down what you intend to do is also a very useful exercise – far better than finding out after months of hard work that you should have used a different strategy, measured an additional variable, or anticipated and catered for a predictable requirement.

Testing hypotheses

When readers turn to the methods section, they are looking for more than details of the apparatus or assay that you used. If your study is descriptive, you will need to answer the questions "Who, what, why, when, and where?" If your research aims to answer a question, you should state exactly what hypothesis was tested – for example, that an intervention should result in a particular effect, such as an increase in survival or improvement in outcome. This is tested by assuming that the null hypothesis is true. The observed results are used to assess how tenable this hypothesis can be – that is, the possibility that the intervention is without effect. The expression of how small this possibility (p value) has to be to disprove the null hypothesis should be stated clearly as the "mission statement" of the study. A study of two antibiotics might compare cure rates: the null hypothesis is that no difference exists, with cure used as the outcome variable. A

p value of less than 0·05 (out of a total probability of 1) implies that values less than this will make the null hypothesis untenable. Many papers merely say, adequately, "$p < 0.05$ was considered significant."

The other side of the coin of probability, which is often neglected, is the *power* of the study. Readers should not be encouraged to believe that, if the null hypothesis has survived attempts to destroy its credibility, no difference probably exists between the groups. This negative outcome may be true or false: you have not shown that your methods are sufficient to test the null hypothesis. Firstly, a true difference may be present, but it might only be small. Secondly, a difference may exist, but the measurements might be variable enough to swamp the effect. In both cases, a small "signal-to-noise" ratio is present. Your methods should, if possible, give an estimate of the power of the study to detect what you are looking for, so that the reader can assess the possibility of a false negative result. This is the β error. The value you choose may depend on factors such as the precision of the answer needed and the practical consequences of an incorrect conclusion, but it is often taken as 0·2, which implies a *power* of 0·8 to avoid a false negative result. In practice, the power of a study depends on the size of the effect, the variability of the data, and the number of observations.

Always state clearly the *a priori* hypotheses – if only to be sure that you collect appropriate and relevant data and do the correct statistical tests.

Statistics

Give the exact tests used to analyse the data statistically, and include an appropriate reference if the test is not well known. If a computer was used, give the type of computer, the software, and the version of the software. The choice of statistical test depends on the type of data. It may not be clear before the data are collected whether parametric tests can be used, in which case the *a priori* tests should be non-parametric.

Design

The study design can often be described with a few well chosen words, particularly if it is a description of the layout of

---

Box 3.1 What to include in the methods section

How the study was designed

- Keep the description brief
- Say how randomisation was done
- Use names to identify parts of a study sequence

How the study was carried out

- Describe how the participants were recruited and chosen
- Give reasons for excluding participants
- Consider mentioning ethical features
- Give accurate details of materials used
- Give exact drug dosages
- Give the exact form of treatment and accessible details of unusual apparatus

How the data were analysed

- Use a *p* value to disprove the null hypothesis
- Give an estimate of the power of the study (the likelihood of a false negative – the β error)
- Give the exact tests used for statistical analysis (chosen *a priori*)

---

groups or events. The groups may be *independent,* allocated to different treatments, and the design is often *parallel,* with each group receiving a different treatment and all groups being entered at the same time. In this case, comparisons will be between groups. Participants who receive different treatments may be *paired* to reduce the effects of confounding variables, such as weight or sex. The effects of a treatment on each participant may be assessed before and after; such comparisons are *within subject.* The simplest study design is a *randomised parallel design*, with a comparison of outcome between groups.

Always state clearly how randomisation was done, because this is a crucial part of many clinical trials. The method used should be stated explicitly in this section. Specific aspects such as blocked randomisation (to obtain roughly similar group sizes) and stratification (to obtain a balance of confounding variables, such as age or sex, in each group) must be described. Authors often choose wrong forms of randomisation, such as alternate cases, unit number, date of birth, and so on. Correct methods involve the use of random number tables or closed envelopes. In a study that involves blind assessment, you may need to describe how the assessor was kept unaware of the treatment allocation. If the adequacy of blinding is important, how will you show that the participants remained unaware of the allocation? Ask the participants to guess after the study is over: is the guess rate better than that expected by chance alone?

A diagram may be helpful if the design of the study is complex or if a complicated sequence of interventions is carried out. You can help readers follow the results by using explicit names for the separate parts of a study sequence; names or even initials to indicate groups or events are preferable to calling them 3, 4, 5, and so on.

Participants and materials

Readers want to know how the participants were recruited and chosen. Healthy, non-pregnant (probably male) volunteers may not reflect the clinical circumstances of many occasions in which a drug is used. Try to give an indication of what disease states have been excluded and how these diseases were defined and diagnosed. What medication leads to exclusion from the study? Alcohol and tobacco use can alter drug responses, and it is tempting to exclude participants who drink and smoke, but the results in such cases would be less applicable to clinical practice. A list of the inclusion and exclusion criteria set out in the ethics application form may be helpful.

Although most journals indicate that ethical approval is a prerequisite for acceptance, some ethical features of the study design may need to be mentioned. For example, you may need to describe some of the practical problems of obtaining informed consent or a satisfactory comparative treatment. Keep a note of eligible participants who are approached and decline to take part: are they different from the participants who agree to the study?

In a laboratory study, details such as the source and strain of animals, bacteria, or other biological material, or the raw materials used are necessary to allow comparisons to be made with other studies and to allow others to repeat the study you have described. Give exact drug dosages (generic name, chemical formula if not well known, and proprietary preparation used, if relevant) and how you prepared solutions, with their precise concentrations.

The exact form of treatment used has to be described in a way that allows replication. If the methods, devices, or techniques are widely known or can be looked up in a standard text – for example, the random zero sphygmomanometer or a Vitalograph spirometer – further information is unnecessary. Similarly, a widely used apparatus, such as the Fleisch pneumotachograph, does not require further description, but less well known apparatus should be described by giving the name, type, and manufacturer.

Methods that are likely to be uncommon or unique should be described fully or an adequate reference to the method should be provided. Readers object if a reference of this sort is only to an abstract or a limited description in a previous paper. If in doubt, provide details and indicate how the methods were validated.

The apparatus used must be described in sufficient detail to allow the reader to be confident of the results reported. Is the apparatus appropriate, sensitive enough, specific in its measurement, reproducible, and accurate? Each aspect may need to be considered separately. For example, bathroom scales may fulfil all of these criteria when used to estimate human body weight, as long as they have been checked and calibrated recently. On the other hand, an inadequate chemical assay may be non-specific because it responds to substances other than its target, gives different results when the same sample is tested twice (poor reproducibility), or gives results that consistently are different from the value expected when tested against a standard substance (poor accuracy). The method may not detect low concentrations (insufficient sensitivity).

The methods used to standardise, calibrate, and assess the linearity and frequency response of the measuring devices used may need to be described. Such characteristics should be given when high fidelity measurements are reported. Do not merely repeat the manufacturer's data for accuracy of a piece of apparatus, particularly if it is crucial to the study: the standard used for a calibration must be stated and the results of the calibration quoted. If analogue to digital conversion is done in computerised analysis, an indication of the sampling rate and the accuracy of the sampling procedure is necessary. Similar considerations of adequate description apply to other methods of assessment and follow up, such as questionnaires, which should be validated.

> **Box 3.2 A good methods section can answer these questions**
>
> - Does the text describe what question was being asked, what was being tested, and how trustworthy the measurements of the variable under consideration would be?
> - Were these trustworthy measurements recorded, analysed, and interpreted correctly?
> - Would a suitably qualified reader be able to repeat the experiment in the same way?

Recommended reading

Eger EI. A template for writing a scientific paper. *Anesth Analg* 1990;**70**:91–6.

Moher D, Schulz KF, Altman DG, for the CONSORT group. The CONSORT statement: revised recommendations for improving the quality of reports of parallel-group randomised trials. *Lancet* 2001;**357**:1191–4.

Grimes DA, Schulz KF. Descriptive studies: what they can and cannot do. *Lancet* 2002;**359**:145–9.

4: The results

HANS-JOACHIM PRIEBE

The results section answers the question "What was found?" It reports the results of the investigation(s) described in the methods section, and it usually does not contain interpretation of data or statements that require referencing. It is composed of words (they tell the story), tables (that summarise the evidence), illustrations (that highlight the main findings), and statistics (that support the statements).

Pay special attention to two pieces of general advice. Firstly, *keep the results section as brief and uncluttered as possible*. The reader must be able to see the wood for the trees. Report only the results that are relevant to the question and hypothesis posed in the introduction section. Secondly, *organise the presentation of results*. Design the text as if you were telling the reader a story. Start chronologically and continue logically to the end. Lead the reader through the story by using a mixture of text, tables, and illustrations.

The words

Start the results section by characterising the participants and objects of your study in enough detail for the reader to assess how representative they were and, if more than one group was studied, how comparable they were. You need to confirm that the participants were comparable, even if they were assigned randomly to the groups. If the groups differ in any way, you will have to comment in the discussion section on how the differences might have affected your results. Items under investigation – for example, bacterial species investigated or substance used – should be mentioned at least once, preferably in the first sentence. When you identify individual participants, use A, B, C, etc. or 1, 2, 3, etc. (when more than 26 subjects) rather than the participant's initials. Do not call the characteristics of subjects the "demographics".

Continue the section by presenting the answers to your main questions. Report results that do not support or that even refute your original hypothesis. Such unexpected results may generate new ideas and can avoid unnecessary future studies. Avoid the much dreaded (by editor, assessor, and reader) statement: "The results are presented in tables X–Z and in figures A–C." Such a statement does not contain any relevant information. On the contrary, it leaves the reader searching for the meaningful result.

Address one topic per paragraph – from most important to least important. Preferably, place those results that directly answer the question posed at the beginning of the results section and of successive paragraphs. Start the paragraph with a topic sentence – a sentence that states the topic or message of the paragraph. The topic is what the paragraph is about, and the message is the point the paragraph is making.

Differentiate clearly between results and data. Results are not identical with data. *Data* are factual findings (often numbers) derived from measurements and observations. Data can be raw (for example, all blood pressure measurements during an investigation), summarised (for example, mean and standard deviation), or transformed (for example, percentage of baseline condition). *Results,* in contrast, state the meaning of the data (for example, "Furosemide administered during mechanical ventilation increased urine output").

Data can rarely be listed without stating the result. For example, consider the following statement: "In 14 untreated individuals, the mean blood glucose concentration was 205 ± 10 (SD) mg%. In 16 patients treated with drug X, the mean blood glucose concentration was 105 ± 10 mg%". The implication of the data is not immediately obvious. The reader is forced to draw their own conclusion, which makes it more difficult for them to read and understand.

Consider a revised version of the same results. "The mean blood glucose concentration was 50% lower in the 16 patients treated with drug X than in the 14 untreated individuals [105 ± 10 (SD) v 205 ± 10 mg%, $p < 0.001$]". This sentence states both the data and the results. The reader now receives immediate information on the direction ("was lower"), the magnitude

("50%"), and the likelihood of a chance finding ("$p < 0.001$") of the observed difference.

Emphasise important results by omitting data from the text, condensing the results, using a result as a topic sentence, putting the most important results at the beginning of a paragraph, and subordinating less important information. Remember that having to sort through a lot of data in the text makes for difficult reading, so data (especially when numerous) are often presented in tables and figures. Avoid duplicating data that are depicted in tables and figures in the text. If several variables change in the same direction, report the resulting change for all variables once rather than the same change variable by variable.

Do not use table headings or figure legends as topic sentences. State the results directly and cite (in parentheses) figures and tables after the first mention of results relevant to the figure or table. For example, consider the following statement: "Systemic haemodynamic data are summarised in Figure 3. Inhalational agent X (1·5 MAC) decreased cardiac output, systemic blood pressure, systemic vascular resistance, and heart rate". The first sentence repeats a figure legend ("Figure 3, Systemic haemodynamic data") and merely indicates the topic – systemic haemodynamic data. After reading the first sentence, the reader has no idea what message to expect in the figure. Only the second sentence carries a message in which the reader is interested – systemic haemodynamic variables decreased. Furthermore, an entire sentence is wasted just on pointing the reader towards a figure.

Consider the revision: "Inhalational agent X (1·5 MAC) decreased cardiac output, systemic blood pressure, systemic vascular resistance, and heart rate (Figure 3)". After reading this sentence, the reader has a clear expectation when turning to the stated figure – decreases in all haemodynamic variables.

Report the results of discrete events in the *past tense,* because they occurred in the past – (for example, "Inhalational agent X inhibited hypoxic pulmonary vasoconstriction"). Report results of a descriptive nature in the *present tense,* because the described state continues to be true. When comparing results, use "than" not "compared with". For example, the statement "X was decreased compared with Y" is ambiguous. It can mean "X was lower than Y", "X decreased more than Y", or "X decreased but Y remained unchanged". State unambiguously what you mean to say.

Be precise in your choice of words. The implication of "We were unable to identify the existence of substance X in material Y" is clearly different from "No substance X was found in material Y". The first statement addresses the issue of ability and implies that substance X may actually exist in material Y but, for whatever reason (like inadequate sensitivity of method), you were not able to identify it. The second statement addresses the issue of actuality and implies that no substance X is present in material Y and thus would not be detected whatever technique was used. Choose the verb according to whether you want to address ability or actuality.

Similarly, the implication of the statement "Substance X *did not* decrease systemic vascular resistance" is clearly different from that of "Substance X *failed to* decrease systemic vascular resistance". "Failed" implies that you actually had expected a decrease in systemic vascular resistance. "Did not" implies no such *a priori* expectation. "Did not decrease" is the usual preferred form used to describe results.

Avoid the use of qualitative words such as "markedly" and "significantly". The reader cannot judge the actual magnitude of a "marked" decrease in systemic blood pressure. Unless accompanied by quantitative data (such as percentage changes) in text, tables or figures, qualitative descriptions are subject to individual judgement. Furthermore, the word "significant" has become a synonym for "statistically significant" and thus can no longer be used interchangeably with "markedly". The wording "Systemic blood pressure decreased significantly" asks for statistical data to support such a statement.

Tables and illustrations: general considerations

Keep in mind that many readers tend to skip the text or read only part of it. They prefer looking at tables and illustrations. It is important therefore that tables and illustrations have strong visual impact, are informative and easy to comprehend, and can stand alone. Readers must be able to interpret them without needing to refer to the text or to other figures and tables. This requires careful design, informative legends for figures, and informative titles and footnotes for tables.

Tables and illustrations should follow a sequence that clearly relates to the text and tells the story of the paper. Design figures and tables and figure legends and footnotes in parallel, so as to prepare the reader for the next table or illustration. Use identical names of variables, units of measurements, and abbreviations in text, tables, and illustrations.

Use the fewest tables and illustrations needed to tell the story. Do not duplicate data in tables and illustrations. It is acceptable to summarise data in tables or illustrations, and to present primary evidence (for example, a single recording of an electroencephalogram) in a separate figure.

Strictly follow the journal's "Instructions to authors". Should you have the misfortune to have your paper refused by one journal, check the instructions and modify the paper before submitting to a second journal. Remember editors and assessors may not look kindly on material that is obviously in the format of another journal.

The tables

In the results section, tables present data that support results. In this context, they serve two main purposes: to present individual data for all subjects and objects studied or to make a point by presenting summary data (for example, means with standard deviations). Each table should deal with a specific problem.

All tables are basically structured the same way, with four main parts: title, column headings, body, and footnotes. Keep the *title* brief, and ensure that it relates clearly to the content of the table. Use identical key terms in the title and column headings, or use a category term (for example, "Effects of inhalational anaesthetic X on systemic haemodynamics") in the title rather than repeating several column headings (for example, "Effects of inhalational anaesthetic X on arterial blood pressure, central venous pressure, cardiac output, and systemic vascular resistance").

The *column headings* consist of headings that identify the items listed in the columns below, subheadings (if required), and units of measurement (if required). Keep column headings brief. For experiments that have independent and dependent variables, the independent variable is in the left column, and the dependent variable in the right column. The sample size (n) can form an additional type of column heading and column.

A table with many dependent variables would become too wide for a page if dependent variables were listed across the top. Placing standard deviations, standard errors of the mean, confidence intervals, or ranges below the mean may solve this problem in some but not all cases. In this instance, consider switching the position of independent and dependent variables. The dependent variables then would be listed down the first column on the left, and the independent variables across the top.

Use *subheadings* to subdivide a heading into further categories. List (mostly in parentheses) the units of measurement after or below the name of the variable in the column heading. Do not repeat them after each value. Use the International System of Units (SI) abbreviations for units of measurement. Make an effort to use units of measurement that avoid listing numerous zeros (for example, "28 km" rather than "28 000 m"). However, avoid the use of multipliers in column headings (for example, "$\times 10^4$") as a means of eliminating zeros. Multipliers are confusing: is the reader supposed to multiply by 10^4 or has the author already done so?

The *body of the table* consists of columns (vertically listed items and data) and rows (horizontally listed items and data). The column on the left lists the items (usually the independent variables) for which data are listed, and the columns on the right list the corresponding data.

Placement of standard deviations can be difficult, especially in the case of several columns. If placed to the right of the mean, reading and comparison of standard deviations across rows are hindered. Likewise, if the standard deviations are placed below the mean, reading and comparison along rows are hindered. If you prefer the reader to make crosswise comparisons, then place the standard deviations below the mean. If you think that lengthwise comparisons are more informative, then place the standard deviations next to the mean. Placing the standard deviations below the mean has the advantage of reducing the width of the table. If you remain unsatisfied with either solution, consider putting the standard deviations in parentheses instead of using ±.

Use the fewest decimal places needed to convey the precision of the measurement. Use the same number of decimal places in means and standard deviations. In each column, align the data on the decimal point (irrespective of whether or not a decimal point is present) and on the ± (for example, when data are presented as mean ± standard deviations).

Tables are a visual medium, so indicate statistically significant differences between data by placing symbols (for example, asterisks (*)) after values that are different, and then define the symbols in the footnote. Do not place symbols after control values or between two values. Adding a separate column of *p* values is not advantageous, because symbols have a greater visual impact and add less bulk to the body of the table. You do not need to identify non-significant differences. As much as a * in a column of aligned numbers is a clear signal of a statistically significant difference, so the absence of a * is a clear signal for the lack of such difference. In addition, NS (for "not significant") is not informative, because the *p* value could have been 0·06 or 0·9.

Usually, a table should include enough data to make it more efficient than listing the numbers in the text. At the same time, it should be small and concise enough to be easily readable. If you have only a small amount of data, list the values in the text. If a table is too large, delete unnecessary columns (for example, a column of *p* values) and rows; avoid repetition of information; keep titles, headings, and subheadings brief; use abbreviations (and explain them in the footnotes); and consider splitting one excessively large table into two smaller tables.

Although certain aspects of table format differ between journals, some generally accepted standards exist. Three horizontal lines are usually used to separate parts of the table: one above the column headings, one below the column headings, and one below the data (to separate the body of the table from the footnotes). In tables with subheadings, short horizontal lines are used to group the subheadings under the respective heading. Avoid (unless requested by a journal's instructions to authors) the use of additional horizontal (between row) and vertical (between column) lines because they give the table a cluttered appearance.

If you want the reader to look at changes, remember that most readers in the Western World read naturally from left to right, not from top to bottom. The results should thus be presented in columns in which the changes run from the

Table 4.1 Heart rate, blood pressure and cardiac output responses

Condition	Heart rate	Systolic BP	Diastolic BP	Cardiac output
Awake	71 ± 10	130 ± 12	84 ± 9	4·264 ± 0·692
Anaesthesia	69 ± 7	112 ± 10	69 ± 8	3·575 ± 0·588
Sternotomy	93 ± 12	177 ± 17	106 ± 13	4·471 ± 0·934
Anaesthesia	79 ± 9	127 ± 12	76 ± 10	3·986 ± 0·765

Table 4.2 Cardiovascular responses to induction of anaesthesia and sternotomy

	Induction of Anaesthesia		Sternotomy	
	Before	After	During	After
Heart rate	71 ± 10	69 ± 7	93 ± 12*	79 ± 9
(beats/min)	(59 – 100)	(53 – 89)	(69 – 130)	(61 – 101)
Systolic BP	130 ± 12	112 ± 10*	177 ± 17*	127 ± 12
(mmHg)	(101 – 148)	(85 – 139)	(121 – 209)	(94 – 149)
Diastolic BP	84 ± 9	69 ± 8*	106 ± 13*	76 ± 10
(mmHg)	(64 – 103)	(50 – 89)	(83 – 131)	(58 – 100)
Cardiac output	4·3 ± 0·7	3·6 ± 0·6*	4·5 ± 0·9	4·0 ± 0·8
(l/min)	(3·1 – 5·9)	(2·6 – 4·9)	(3·0 – 6·1)	(2·9 – 5·2)

Data are means ± SD (range) obtained in 11 patients five minutes before and after induction of anaesthesia, and during and five minutes after sternotomy. BP = blood pressure. *$p < 0.05$ v "before induction of anaesthesia" by ANOVA

left-most column. Often, it helps to present results as percentage changes from the initial value. If you do this, include an initial column of actual data as well.

Tables 4.1 and 4.2 illustrate what is often submitted and how the information can be made to look much better.

Table 4.1 is an example of a poor table. The title does not explain the initiating stimulus to the observed responses. It lists individual haemodynamic variables rather than using a category term. The "condition" is poorly defined. All of the vertical and most of the horizontal grid lines are superfluous. The columns have no indication of the units used. The results for cardiac output show more decimal places than the precision of the measurement justifies. The ± value is not defined (is it standard deviation or standard error of the mean?). No mention is made of the number of participants studied. The changes run from top to bottom rather than from left to right across the page. Abbreviations are not explained. No indication is given of any statistically significant changes.

Consider now a revised version of the same table (Table 4.2).

When considered in combination with the footnote, this table provides all the information needed by the reader. The title describes the initiating stimuli ("Induction of anaesthesia and sternotomy") and uses a category term ("cardiovascular"). The superfluous grid lines are eliminated. Changes run across the table from the left-most column. The subheadings ("Before", "After", "During", and "After") allow clear chronological allocation of observation points. Units of measurement are provided. The asterisks in two columns are a clear signal of a statistically significant difference (the absence is a clear signal for the lack of such a difference). The footnote defines the kind of data, the number of patients studied, the observation points, the abbreviations, the statistical significance level, and the statistics used. This table can now stand on its own. Your reader will be able to obtain all the information they need without having to refer back to the text.

The illustrations

The main purpose of illustrations in the results section is to present evidence that supports the results – either as primary evidence (for example, electrocardiographs or radiographs) or as numerical data (for example, graphs or histograms).

Ensure good readability. Remember that illustrations have to go through a number of processes before appearing in print. With each process, some detail will be lost, so make sure the quality of your originals is as good as possible. Check legibility by reducing the figure to publication size with a photocopier. The smallest letter should be at least 1·5 mm high. Symbols must be large enough to be identified easily. Emphasise important information by using different line weights. Make each figure deliver a clear message. Only some key points can be given here, so use Tufte's books (see the recommended reading list), which are excellent guides as to what can and should be done.

Present primary evidence when this is the type of data you have or when you want to show the quality of your data acquisition. For example, a paper reporting an investigation on coronary blood flow, in addition to summarising your data in numerical form (for example, in graphs or tables), could show a representative coronary blood flow recording. Select the best quality recording for reproduction.

Label your illustrations adequately. The extent of labelling depends on the readership. The more general the readership, the more labelling usually is required. Labels include arrows, arrowheads, letters, numbers, and symbols. Define the labels in the figure legend. Use the fewest, briefest, and smallest labels possible.

Figure legends

A figure legend is a descriptive statement that is placed next to the figure. It is essential to make the figure understandable without the reader needing to refer to the text. The type of figure will determine the content of the figure legend, which typically consists of up to four parts: a brief title, experimental details, various definitions (for example, of symbols or abbreviations), and statistical information.

Keep the title brief, use the same key terms that you use in the figures and text, and avoid the use of abbreviations. Where appropriate, provide just enough experimental detail to allow the reader to understand the figure. Define symbols or line patterns by redrawing them in the figure legend. Make sure that the patterns in the legend match the patterns in illustrations. If identical symbols or abbreviations are used in several figures, define them the first time they occur and then refer the reader to the legend that contains the definitions.

The statistical information required in the figure legend depends on the type of illustration. Information for graphs should include whether data represent individual, mean, or median values; whether error bars represent standard deviations (SD), standard errors of the mean (SEM), confidence intervals (CI), or ranges; and the sample size (n). For bar graphs, state which values were compared by statistical analysis, the significance value (p value), and possibly the statistical test you used. Avoid writing "$n = 11$", as such statements may be ambiguous; be more specific – for example, write "11 blood samples", "11 measurements" or "11 rats". In addition to this standard structure of a figure legend, the legend can point to an unusual or interesting finding.

When you use photographs of patients, you must obtain written, informed consent before an individual's photograph is taken and published. Cover facial features whenever possible. Use A, B, etc., not initials, when you need to refer to a patient.

When using polygraph recordings, eliminate grid lines and add vertical and horizontal scales. Make sure that scales and scale markers are absolutely accurate. Label each scale marker with the appropriate unit. Use the SI abbreviations for units of measurement.

Many types of graphs are available, so carefully choose the graph that best represents your data. In line graphs, the independent variable (for example, time) is conventionally on the x-axis and the dependent variable (for example, blood pressure) on the y-axis. If the scale is linear, tick marks and scale numbers must be spaced at equal distances and intervals, respectively, starting where the axes meet. In a bar graph, the axis must include zero, otherwise, the differences between bars are obscured. As the baseline is not an axis, so no line or tick marks are needed along the baseline.

Republishing figures

You need to first obtain permission from the copyright holder (usually the publisher) – this is a legal requirement. You should also obtain permission from the author, as common courtesy. Standard permission forms are available from publishers.

Give attribution to the source and the publisher. Cite the reference in the figure legend and state that you have permission for republication. Credit is always given at the very end of a figure legend. Attribution can read as follows: "From Laver et al. (1981), with permission", or "From ref. 10, with permission from the *British Journal of Anaesthesia*". When you have modified an original illustration, the attribution could read: "Redrawn from Laver et al. (1981); reproduced with permission".

The statistics

Statistics must accompany data. Many papers suffer because the statistics are badly presented. Obviously, many statistical tests exist – conventional as well as esoteric. Choose the test most appropriate for your data analysis. Decide on which statistical test to use when planning your study. Do not take the data of your finished study to your local statistician to see what can be made of them – that is a waste of everyone's time.

Follow some general rules. As data are mostly restricted to tables and figures, that is where you should include most statistical data. Specify the type of statistic, the sample size (n), and the probability value for a test of statistical significance (p value). When normally distributed data have been analysed statistically, report the mean and a statistic that indicates the variation from the mean (for example, the standard deviation or the range). When non-normally distributed data have been analysed statistically, report the median and the interquartile range (the range between the 25th and the 75th percentiles).

When you list statistical details in the text, follow some conventional rules. Mean and standard deviation are usually written as "11·4 ± 0·8 (SD) kg." The conventional way to write data that are being compared statistically is: "Body weight increased more in group A than in group B [13·2 ± 1·9 (SD) v 9·4 ± 0·9 kg in eight patients, $p < 0.02$]". This statement contains five types of statistical information: the mean ("13·2" and "9·4 kg"), the standard deviation ("1·9" and "0·9"), specification of the statistic used to describe the variation from the mean ("SD"), the sample size (n) ("8 patients"), and the probability value of significance ("$p < 0.02$"). Usually, you should provide all five types of statistical information; however, if any of these statistical parameters apply to all data (for example, SD and sample size), you only need to describe the complete statistical details when you list the data the first time and can omit thereafter those that apply to all data. If you decide to report the confidence interval, the statement can be rewritten as follows: "Body weight increased more in group A than in group B [13·2 ± 1·9 (SD) v 9·4 ± 0·9 kg in eight patients; 95% confidence interval for the difference = 1·8 – 5·2 kg, $p < 0.02$]".

When you provide p values, you should list the actual p values not only for those differences considered statistically significant (for example, $p < 0.02$), but also for differences not considered significant (for example, $p > 0.6$ or $p = 0.55$). By restricting the information to statements like "$p > 0.05$" or "$p = \text{NS}$", you restrict the reader's ability to interpret the data accurately: a p value of 0.06 does not exclude the possibility of a statistically significant difference as strongly as a p value of > 0.9.

Do not list data to a greater degree of accuracy than that of the measurement. For example, if you can measure cardiac output with an accuracy of only $\pm 10\%$, do not quote values for individual results to three decimal places. Make sure that any change described as statistically significant is greater than the error of your measurement. Be particularly careful with calculated values: the errors of the original measurements add up alarmingly.

Take care when you look at associations between variables. Statistical significance needs to indicate how much of an association can be attributed to the dependency of one variable on another and how much is due to chance. Be careful with extrapolation, and do not confuse association with causation.

Statistical presentation is always a problem – too much information, too little space. Present enough information for the intelligent reader to believe what you are saying. Remember: usually, neither your readers, nor your assessors, are expert statisticians. If your statistical tests are too esoteric, be prepared for a lengthy discussion before publication.

Conclusion

The results section is the easiest to write. The introduction has defined the questions and the methods the means of getting the answers. Decide during the design stage of your study how the results will be presented. Apart from filling in the actual data in the tables and placing the actual dots and lines in the figures, you could almost write the results as you start the investigation. Remember to follow the general design of the results section: the text should tell the story, the tables will summarise the evidence, the illustrations will show the highlights, and the statistics should support your statements. Keep it all straightforward – and always *keep the reader in mind*.

Recommended reading

Zeiger M. *Essentials of writing biomedical research papers.* New York: McGraw-Hill, 2000. (An outstanding guide to good scientific writing that contains numerous exercises.)

Huth EJ. *Writing and publishing in medicine.* Baltimore: Williams & Wilkens, 1999. (An excellent book about the process of writing and publishing.)

O'Connor M. *Writing successfully in science.* London: Chapman & Hall, 1991. (An excellent guide to the topic.)

Tufte ER. *The visual display of quantitative information.* Cheshire, CT: Graphics Press, 1983. (This book shows what is too often done and what can be done.)

Tufte ER. *Visual explanations.* Cheshire, CT: Graphics Press, 1997. (This is a guide on how to use graphics and to get your point across.)

5: Discussion

HARVEY MARCOVITCH

Structure

By now you have answered three questions: "Why did we do it?" (Introduction), "What did we do?" (Methods), and "What did we find?" (Results). It is now time to put all of this into context by dealing with a fourth question: "So what?"

When you are considering what to write, keep in the forefront of your mind the message you wish to put across to your readers. Otherwise, the distinct risk is that your discussion will meander into historical byways and blind alleys. In addition, keep as closely as you can to the usual format of a discussion section in a scientific journal. When you look through medical journals you will find that, in general, this comes to seven or eight paragraphs of three or four sentences each. You should check a few issues of your target journal to make sure it is not unusual in this respect. Remember that a paragraph consists of a key sentence, followed by subsidiary sentences that put flesh onto its bones. Each paragraph should lead logically onto the next until you give your conclusion.

Getting started

You can start in various ways. Firstly, you could begin with a summary of the field of enquiry. For example, investigators who measured blood lead in children with behavioural problems began their discussion with the sentence: "Lead, a known neurotoxin, has been shown to affect the cognition and development of young children."

Alternatively, you can tempt readers to continue reading by pointing out why your study is special – along the lines of: "This study is unique, case-controlled, and evaluated the outcome of those treated with prophylactic antibiotics for at least six months." If the journal's reviewers have put you on the defensive, you might wish to pre-empt criticism: "This study, like most dealing with child abuse, faces a major obstacle – that of bias generated by denial."

Some authors start the discussion section with their main finding as the first sentence, rather like how newspapers put across a report's message in the opening sentence. For example, in a paper, "The impact of HIV-1 on laryngeal airway obstruction in children", the discussion might begin: "In this study, HIV-1 infection was present in half of the patients admitted with laryngeal airway obstruction, creating a substantial demand for scarce ICU [intensive care unit] resources. More usually, scientific authors mimic the IMRAD [Introduction, Methods, Results, And Discussion] convention in this section, keeping readers in suspense by reserving their main message for the first sentence of the final paragraph. This often begins: "We conclude …" or "This study found …". In a paper such as that above the last paragraph might be used to remind readers that the data could be used in future cohort studies and that HIV infection is not a contraindication to patients receiving care in intensive care units – two subsidiary messages that arose from the study.

Summarising the literature

Whichever way you start your discussion, try not to repeat what you have already stated in the introduction to your paper. You rather should place your findings in the context of what is already known about the topic. This implies that, before putting pen to paper or fingers to keyboard, you should conduct a careful and thorough trawl of the databases – preferably, of course, before starting your research project. Do not be tempted to quote papers you have not read (probably the major reason for the high error rate in reference lists). You should quote findings that contradict your own, as well as those that support them, and analyse what might have caused any disparity.

A common weakness, especially of inexperienced authors, is to attempt a detailed critique of everything that has gone before. The result is likely to be an overlong paper that will fail to hold readers' (and more importantly reviewers' and editors') attention. Before writing this section, therefore, sort your references into those with an important message and those without. Discard the latter – wondering briefly why the editors of the journals in which they were published failed to do so themselves. Decide which of the remainder seem to have involved the strongest methods and make them the centrepiece of your historical review. Where you are convinced a previous publication is not sound, it is important to give the reasons why you believe your own data are firmer. This is essential if the quoted reference is attractive superficially or is cited often.

Stating your case

Next you should refer to your own results (without repeating them in detail) in terms of what they add to the existing body of knowledge and how they advance understanding of the subject. You should refer honestly to any doubts you or others might have about the validity of your data, especially with reference to confounding factors and to any wide confidence intervals exposed in statistical analyses quoted in the results. Frequently, this is one area where good reviewers can help authors improve their paper.

You should deal with the practical lessons to be learned (if any) – such as how your findings might alter matters such as diagnostic precision, clinical care, or epidemiological understanding – depending on the nature of your research.

Some journals, such as the *BMJ*, may ask you to summarise this section in a box along the lines of "What is already known on this topic" and "What this study adds."

Finishing off

Try to end with a bang not a whimper. As an editor who critically considers submissions, I am always disappointed when the final sentence or two reveal that the study provides little of use for the reader to take away. Albert, who teaches medical writing, pointed out that nearly all scientific papers end in three ways: "perhaps … possibly", "more research is needed," and "here's another problem solved".[1] If you can manage the last of these endings, your paper should be a winner. The middle option is not to be despised, as many papers beg more questions than they answer. If this is indeed what you conclude, however, your paper will have a much stronger message if it points the way to what sort of research is needed – as long as it doesn't sound too much like a grant application. The weakest papers are those that end with the first alternative. This is not to say that negative findings are less important than positive findings: discovering that your data do not support the original hypothesis is a thoroughly justifiable conclusion, but to be unable to state whether or not the findings do support the hypothesis is not.

Avoiding pitfalls

The most disappointing papers are those in which the conclusions are not backed up by the data. It is not unusual to begin a research project with the hope of finding a particular answer; if some data let you down, however, do not succumb to the temptation to gloss over them in the interests of your desired conclusion. This is always a mistake: in Greek mythology, Procrustes performed ruthless orthopaedic surgery on hapless travellers who did not fit his only bed. In clinical practice, patients may face disaster if a doctor decides on a diagnosis and then bends the signs or symptoms to back it up, rather than retesting his hypothesis as each new piece of information arises. When an author writes papers, the first of these approaches risks disapproval by reviewers and rejection by editors. Such papers that nonetheless pass through the net tend to be criticised repeatedly by others – or worse, are not cited at all.

Editorial committees groan when yet another author confuses association with cause and effect. Remember, if you enter a large enough number of variables into a regression analysis, at least one will prove statistically significant at a 5% level. This does not mean that it is true or that reviewers and editors will be convinced.

Get the message across

After you have written your first draft, ask yourself (or a friend) whether you have got the message across. Make sure your argument progresses logically, with each paragraph leading the reader step by step towards your conclusion. If this does not happen, you will lose many readers on the way, as they turn over to something that catches and holds their attention. One way of checking whether you have done this is to look at your manuscript and underline each sentence that is key in the advancement of the argument. Most should appear at the start of paragraphs, but some are likely to be at the end. If they appear in the middle, the structure of your paragraphs is wrong. If large blocks of print are not underlined, they are likely to be redundant and should be the first to go when you exceed the desired word count.* This fate is most likely to befall sections inserted against your better judgement by co-authors or unthinkingly by you at the behest of reviewers.

Adding the extras

Beneath your discussion, you may need to enter acknowledgements to those who enabled the project to be carried out successfully. This should include whoever funded the research – although in some journals this information is published separately, such as in the scholar's margin that contains the authors' names or institutions. This is particularly important if there is any risk of you having an actual or potential competing interest – for example, in a study funded by a pharmaceutical company. Even where a journal does not ask specifically for a declaration of interest you should insert one.

Polite authors thank the patients or clients who participated in the trial (who should never be referred to as "subjects"), as well as those who provided technical or statistical help. This should remind you to reconsider whether their contribution was sufficient to recategorise them as authors. You may wish to acknowledge secretarial help, but probably only if it has gone well beyond the call of duty. Scientific papers are not Hollywood Oscars, so it is rarely necessary to include your devoted spouse, however irritated by late night word processing, or your beloved children, however neglected because of your searching the database. One sycophantic author insisted on including the editor because of his stouthearted translation of the paper from Franglais – this is not recommended, as it suggests the possibility of a conflict of interest.

Summary
- Be consistent with target journal's style
- Three ways to start your piece: mini-seminar, main finding, or what's different
- Summarise relevant *important* previous work
- Put your results in context
- Mention doubts, weaknesses, and confounders
- Offer data supported practical advice (if any)
- Three ways of ending: problem solved, more research needed, or uncertainty remains

Reference

1 www.timalbert.co.uk/shortwords_research.html (accessed 10/10/2002).

*The desired word count is that advised in the journal's instructions to authors or, if not included, the mean of several papers randomly chosen from that journal. Many editors prefer shorter rather than longer papers, as their annual pagination budget is limited. This may not apply to electronic publication, as cyberspace is unlimited.

6: Titles, abstracts, and authors

FIONA MOSS

Introduction

Getting a paper published is one thing. Writing a paper that is a "good read" requires additional skill and thought. Professional writers – for example, journalists who write for a living – write for readers. They want their message to get to as many people as possible. Many papers submitted to medical journals are dull, and, on first reading, it is not clear what they are about. Messages are difficult to find and the reader is challenged by dense writing. Only the truly determined – usually people in the same micro-field – make it through to the end. Many papers published in medical journals are read by very few people.

In modern times, a person's academic worth equates with the number of papers they have "authored." They are under pressure to publish, so that papers can be considered for research assessment exercises and academic preferment. Often, the number of papers published is considered more important than their quality, and no marks are awarded for clarity of writing. But editors are readers too. So, a well written paper with a clear message is more likely to get through the editorial process than one that is equally worthy but dull and impenetrable.

Preparation of a research paper is not the same as writing a novel: it is not an exercise in creative writing. Conventions exist for describing the study design, results, and details of statistical analyses, and few ways exist to describe molecular structures or lung function tests. Nevertheless, within the limitations of the form, it is possible to write for the reader with clarity as well as accuracy and without burying the important messages in turgid, jargon-ridden prose. The use of a simple and straightforward style is essential, but being clear

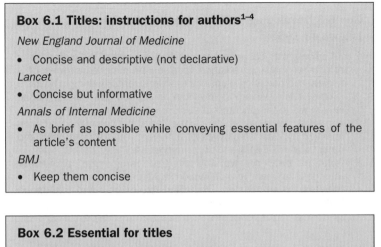

Box 6.1 Titles: instructions for authors[1–4]

New England Journal of Medicine

- Concise and descriptive (not declarative)

Lancet

- Concise but informative

Annals of Internal Medicine

- As brief as possible while conveying essential features of the article's content

BMJ

- Keep them concise

Box 6.2 Essential for titles

- Concise and precise
- Informative and descriptive
- Not misleading or unrepresentative
- Specific – for example, include type of study and numbers (if large)
- Words appropriate for classification
- Interesting not dull

about what the paper is about comes first. So start by making sure that the title and abstract are compelling as well as accurate. Truthfully, many people will not read much else. And unless the title and the abstract can "grab" the reader, they are unlikely to read on.

Titles (Box 6.1)

The title is important. Consider it as the signpost that tells the reader what your paper is about and encourages them to invest time in your paper. Titles must be functional, should be direct, and need not be dull. Use simple language. Be concise, memorable, and informative, with an edge to alert the browsing reader and encourage them to read on, and with just enough detail for the focused reader to recognise the paper for which they have been searching (Box 6.2).

Titles that are too clever or whimsical may briefly interest a browser but be missed by the purposeful reader. Avoid being very short and cryptic, as the words in the title may be used

Box 6.3 Developing a title in four steps (after Lilleyman, 1998)[5]

1 An epidemiological geographically based study of the quantity and effects of ionising radiation received by male employees of a nuclear reprocessing plant and male residents working elsewhere in the same vicinity shows an increased risk of childhood leukaemia in the children of nuclear workers only
2 An epidemiological study of the links between the radiation received by male employees of a nuclear reprocessing plant and other local residents and childhood leukaemia
3 Relation between working at and living near a nuclear reprocessing plant and childhood leukaemia
4 **"Nuclear reprocessing, radiation exposure, and childhood leukaemia: an epidemiological study"**

by electronic search engines to identify and categorise papers. To describe a comparative study of the prevalence of asthma in Birmingham and Hereford as "A tale of two cities" would not work as a signpost for the reader and, given the binary logic of computers, might mean the paper is eventually linked electronically with papers on town planning.

Some tips (Box 6.3)

1 Describe your paper in two or three sentences.
2 Précis these sentences: remove unnecessary occurrences of "as" and "the," as well as any references to the results.
3 Now write a draft title.
4 Review this. Perhaps try the technique of "a title in two parts", for example, giving the main subject and the type of the study. For example, "Improving the repeat prescribing process in a busy general practice: a study using continuous quality improvement methods."
5 Check:

- Is it accurate?
- Is it in any way misleading?
- Does it contain essential key words?
- Is it interesting?

It may be the only part of the paper that will be read, so make sure it encourages the reader to read on.

Abstracts

Abstracts are usually the only part of the paper freely available via electronic search engines and are read by many more people than the rest of the paper. It is crucial, therefore, to sum up your paper in 200–300 words.

Structured abstracts are now the norm for papers that report original research. These provide a format that requires authors to summarise their work systematically by disclosing context, objectives, design, setting, participants, interventions, main outcome measures, results, and conclusions. Structured abstracts thus are informative and help peer reviewers and readers.[6] The abstract format is based on the standard IMRAD (Introduction, Methods, Results, And Discussion) structure of papers, but it is more detailed – for example, design, setting, participants, and interventions are sub-sections of the methods – so writing the abstract should ensure authors include essential detail in the main paper.

Abstract headings vary a little between journals and for different types of research. Not all research includes an intervention, and clinical research needs to describe participants, whereas meta-analyses include data sources and study selection. Unstructured abstracts are often required for papers that do not describe original research.

Structures based on the IMRAD format do not suit all types of work. Quality improvement work that includes repeated cycles of measurement and change cannot be easily expressed in the standard formats. To help authors express what matters in this type of work, the editorial team of *Quality and Safety in Health Care* devised a structure that reflects important aspects of quality improvement work.[7,8] The format includes, for example, strategies for change, lessons learned, and messages for others (see Box 6.4). Although the structure is different, the process and guidance for writing the abstract are the same.

Some tips

1   Start to write the paper by preparing the abstract. This may be the most difficult part of the paper to get right, but doing it first will help you to clarify your messages and make writing the rest of the paper easier.

Box 6.4 Structure for quality improvement reports

Context
- What are the relevant details of staff groups and functions of departments?

Outline of problem
- What were you trying to accomplish?

Key measures for improvement
- What would constitute success in the patient's view?

Process of gathering information
- What methods were used to assess problems?

Analysis and interpretation
- How did this information change your understanding of the problem?

Strategy for change
- What changes were made?
- How were they implemented?
- Who was involved?

Effects of change
- How did this lead to improvement for patients?

Next steps
- What have you learned/achieved?
- How will you take this forward?

---

2 Check:

- Are abstract headings appropriate for the type of research?
- Are they those required for the journal to which you are submitting: for example, background or context, objectives or aims, methods or design, results or outcome, and conclusions or discussion?

3 Check the maximum number of words. This varies between journals, but it usually ranges between 200 and 300 words.

4 Use phrases rather than sentences but maintain coherence and sense. Purple prose with too many adjectives and adjectival clauses has no place in scientific papers, but neither should the language be so terse that it becomes a knotted mass of words.

5   Check whether the abstract makes sense and that you are getting your message across. Ask a colleague who is not involved in the research to read it. Do they understand your message?

6   Check for consistency. The abstract should reflect the paper and describe your message succinctly and accurately. As soon as the paper is written, compare the abstract with the paper. Do the objectives described in the abstract match those in the paper? New words that change the emphasis can appear in the process of pruning e.g. appropriateness is not the same as suitability or usability.

7   Finally, remember that more people read the abstract than the whole paper and that many only read the abstract and may only give it one try.

Authors (or contributors?)

Authors are writers – at least that is the common usage of the word. Rohinton Mistry, Sara Paretsky, and JK Rowling are authors. They write. They create. The Harry Potter books – from idea to manuscript – are the work of JK Rowling. The word author also describes originators or creators other than writers, for example, the author of this plan or the author of congestion charging in London. When used in reference to papers in medical and scientific journals, however, the word author has a meaning that stretches beyond standard usage. Moreover, only rarely is there a single author of a medical paper. Authorship is shared with others. Clearly many authors are neither the originator nor the writer of the paper, but they are all essential to the team, to the development of ideas, to the technical input, to the interpretation of results.

Authorship is a valued commodity that can be given and withdrawn. It can be "gifted" in several ways. Firstly, "back scratching" is when researchers working in related areas in the same unit swap authorships by putting each other on their papers, thus bolstering the number of papers that each has "authored." Secondly, "toadying" is the custom of including, as authors, senior people who have influence but only a tenuous link to the paper – they may have been asked to look at an early draft, although they may not actually have read it. Thirdly, "patronage" involves including as authors those involved solely because of routine administrative or technical tasks – usually, for example, seventh in a list of 10.

Less is known about the dark practice of not including people with a legitimate claim to authorship. Many stories exist, and are told and retold, of colleagues who, despite contributing hugely to all stages of a project, were dropped from the final list of authors. Radiologists regularly complain of being excluded from authorship of case reports that rely on radiographic findings or images. This isn't always dented pride: without their input, case reports sometimes wrongly describe findings.

Defining who should or should not be an author is not straightforward, and editors and researchers sometimes disagree. The Vancouver guidelines state that "each author should have participated sufficiently in the work to take public responsibility for the content" and that authorship credit should be based on substantial contributions to:[9]

1 concept and design or analysis and interpretation of data
2 drafting of the article or revising it critically for important intellectual content
3 final approval of the version to be published.

Authors must meet all three criteria. All other contributions, including data collection, should be mentioned in acknowledgements.[9]

Editors, it seems, are less tolerant than researchers about including people who have contributed technically. Researchers do not like editors to make decisions about who or who should not be considered an author and although they may agree with each of the three "Vancouver criteria," many are unhappy about having to meet all of them.[10] Much is at stake for researchers, because authorship is a sign of academic success.

Contributorship

Being an author gives credit, but it also carries responsibility. In some cases of publication of fraudulent data, co-authors have not accepted responsibility. The many problems with authorship – from gifting and ghosting to fraud and acceptance of responsibility – have led to the suggestion that authorship should be scrapped. Instead, people should be listed as contributors with a clear statement of each person's role, and, importantly, someone should take the role of guarantor of the paper.[11–13]

That suggestion was first made six years ago – in 1997. Authorship and debate about authorship continue, but several journals, including *JAMA*, *BMJ*, and *Lancet*, list each author's contribution. In addition, as one defence against publication of fraudulent work, some journals require one contributor to be identified as the guarantor responsible for the study. The Vancouver group recommends that the guarantor provides a written statement to acknowledge that they accept responsibility for conduct of the study, that they had access to data, and that they controlled the decision to publish.

Conventions of order

The Vancouver guidelines suggest that nothing should be inferred from the order of authors (because conventions between countries, specialties, and research groups differ). Much is assumed, however, and the position of first author is coveted.[14] If more than six authors are involved, many journals include the first three and sum up the rest as "*et al.*" The first author is likely to have been the person who wrote the paper, and the second and third authors are likely to be significant contributors. The last author is usually the heavy weight and is likely to be the guarantor – but not always, hence the need for the clarification provided by contributor lists.

Some tips

- Discuss "contributorship" early on.
- Ask everyone to write down their contribution.
- Agree contributions.
- Establish who is to be guarantor.
- Ensure that all contributors can see raw data.
- Arrange for all contributors to meet to discuss interpretation of data.

- Ensure that all contributors have the opportunity to comment as the paper is drafted.
- Agree order of contributors.
- Agree who should be acknowledged.

References

1 *BMJ* house style. http://bmj.com/advice/stylebook/start.shtml
2 http://www.annals.org/shared/manu_format.html
3 http://www.thelancet.com/
4 *Help for Authors.* http://www.nejm.org/hfa/
5 Lilleyman JS. Titles, Abstracts, Authors. In: *How to Write a Paper.* Second edition. London: BMJ Publishing Group, 1998.
6 Haynes RB, Mulrow CD, Huth EJ, Altman DG, Gardner MJ. More informative abstracts revisited. *Ann Intern Med* 1990;**113**:69–76.
7 Moss F, Thomson R. A new structure for quality improvement reports. *Qual Saf Health Care* 1999;**8**:76.
8 Smith R. Quality improvement reports: a new kind of article. *BMJ* 2000;**321**:1428–9.
9 Uniform requirements for manuscripts to medical journals. http://www.icmje.org/
10 Bhopal R, Rankin J, McColl E, *et al.* The vexed question of authorship: views of researchers in a British medical faculty. *BMJ* 1997;**314**:1009–12.
11 Rennie D, Yank V, Emanuel L. When authorship fails: a proposal to make contributors accountable. *JAMA* 1997:**278**:579–85.
12 Smith R. Authorship is dying: long live contributorship. *BMJ* 1997;**315**:696.
13 Horton R. The signature of responsibility. *Lancet* 1997;**350**:5–6.
14 Chambers R, Boath E, Chambers S. The A–Z of authorship: analysis of influence of initial letter of surname on order of authorship. *BMJ* 2001; **323**:1460–1.

7: References

SIMON HOWELL

Introduction

The references of your paper are the foundation on which your work is built. They provide the scientific background that justifies the research you have undertaken and the methods you have used. They provide the context in which your research should be interpreted. They should not be collected as an afterthought when your research project is complete. A literature search and reading of the relevant references should be the starting points of any research project. Undertaking research to confirm the findings of another study of course is entirely justified. It is futile, however, to invest many hours of time and effort in a research project, only to discover that your findings are well established facts that have been confirmed in many previous studies. In some cases, such a study could be argued to be unethical, in that it subjects animals, volunteers, or patients to research that leads to no new knowledge or understanding.

Searching the literature

The advent of electronic bibliographic databases of the medical and scientific literature has transformed the exercise of performing a literature search. These databases are generally accessible via the internet and have stored within them the details of many thousands of references from hundreds of journals. The records are usually indexed in various ways to facilitate searching and provide tools that allow simple and more sophisticated interrogation of the database. A search that previously would have required many hours in a library ploughing through the large volumes of the *Index Medicus* can now be completed in a few minutes sitting at a computer. The speed and range of these electronic tools is such, however, that the searchers may find themselves swamped by an avalanche of citations. Some thought and practice is needed to get the best from these powerful tools.

Many bibliographic databases cover various aspects of the medical and scientific literature and may be relevant to the medical researcher. Probably the two most widely used are Medline and EMBASE. Medline is produced by the United States National Library of Medicine and covers the fields of medicine, nursing, dentistry, veterinary medicine, the healthcare system, and the preclinical sciences. It contains over 11 million citations that date back to the mid 1960s. EMBASE, the Excerpta Medica database, is produced by Elsevier Science. About 30% of journals that may be searched through EMBASE also appear in Medline, but EMBASE has a more European emphasis than Medline and is useful for identifying citations in non-English language journals. EMBASE has a strong emphasis on drugs, pharmacology, and toxicology, and it is valuable for identifying citations in these areas. To complete a comprehensive search, you probably need to examine both databases. For clinical research, and especially for those planning a clinical trial or systematic review, a visit to the Cochrane Library (http://www.update-software.com) is probably essential. At the core of the Cochrane Library is its database of systematic reviews. It also contains a number of other valuable resources, including the Cochrane Central Register of Controlled Trials and the Cochrane Methodology Register.

A large number of other databases are available (Box 7.1). Among these, CINAHL covers the nursing literature, PsycINFO is a useful gateway to the psychological and psychiatric literature and HMIC is a valuable resource for research in health management. It is easy to be overwhelmed by the extent and complexity of what is available. Start by searching the "mainstream" databases discussed above and, if you find it is essential to venture more widely, seek the advice of a medical librarian. They will be able to tell you what databases are available locally, which may be relevant, and how best to search them.

The various databases have a number of search interfaces. Among the most widely used are PubMed and Ovid. The former gives access to the Medline database and is an internet gateway maintained by the United States National Library of

> **Box 7.1 Common databases**
>
> Allied and Complementary Medicine Database (AMED)
> Applied Social Sciences Index and Abstracts (ASSIA)
> British Nursing Index (BNI)
> Cumulative Index to Nursing and Allied Health Literature (CINAHL)
> Digital Dissertations
> Health Management Information Consortium Databases (HMIC)
> National Research Register (NRR) (an NHS research register)
> Popline (a population database)
> PsycINFO (database of psychological abstracts)
> Toxline (bibliographic database for toxicology)

Medicine. It can be found at http://www.ncbi.nlm.nih.gov/ PubMed. PubMed has the merits of being freely available on the internet and having a particularly user friendly interface. It only provides access to one bibliographic database, however. Ovid is a commercial organisation that provides access to a wide range of bibliographic databases including Medline and EMBASE. The precise databases available via Ovid vary from subscriber to subscriber. The user interface is rather more complex than that provided by PubMed, but it is a powerful tool for complex searches. Ovid also has the merit that it includes a range of other databases for searching, as well as Medline and EMBASE. Ask your local medical library for details of which databases are available and how to access them.

To conduct basic searches with these databases is not difficult. The user is provided with a box into which to type keywords, authors' names, or the title of a journal. Such a query may produce the response that no matches were found, but more frequently, a list of citations is returned. This may be several hundred references in length and could include material that is highly relevant, as well as citations that are not relevant at all. For this reason, you should gain some skill in searching these databases, as time invested in doing this will be repaid many times over in the future. Ovid provides extensive help files that explain how to get the best from the search engine. PubMed has help files and an extremely good interactive tutorial that provides an excellent introduction to how to use the database.

All entries in Medline are indexed with a detailed set of medical subject headings or MeSH terms, over 15 000 of which cover the whole range of medical subjects. Most terms are associated with a series of subheadings, and these headings and subheadings can be qualified further to focus on areas of special interest, such as epidemiology or therapeutics. A search based on MeSH terms is likely to be more successful than a general query. PubMed provides a browser of MeSH terms, so you can identify and use relevant MeSH terms. In Ovid, the same strategy may be applied by asking the search engine to map the search terms to the relevant database headings or thesaurus. EMBASE uses a similar set of subject headings, which may again be accessed using the mapping facility provided by Ovid. If you are unsure of the relevant MeSH terms or subject headings for your search, use the database to identify a reference you know to be relevant and note the terms used to index that reference.

Both Ovid and PubMed allow the history of the current search strategy to be examined and the search to be refined. The "cubby" facility in PubMed and the "save current search facility" of Ovid allow details of the search to be saved, so it can be run again at a later date. Other tools allow limits to be set on what citations are returned by a given search: for example, a date range can be identified, the type of reference to be returned can be selected (for example, review or randomised controlled trial), studies of animals or of humans may be requested, and the search may be limited to English language references only.

A particularly useful feature of PubMed is the facility that allows searchers to find references that cover the same material as a given citation. Beside each reference identified in a PubMed search is a link labelled "Related articles". Clicking this link initiates a search that identifies references that cover the same material as the original citation.

Apart from a formal search strategy with medical subject headings, often it is useful to search for papers written by known workers in the field of interest. When you identify references through Medline, you may discover that, in some cases, the title carries the suffix "see comments" and links to correspondence about the paper. Such correspondence may offer useful pointers to the interpretation of the paper and may be an indicator of current debate in the field of interest.

In both Ovid and PubMed, the abstracts of the references found may be displayed. You should scan these online and mark relevant ones to download and print. (The alternative is to print the references and read them offline, but you could end up printing out an unconscionably large number of references.) The "clipboard" facility of PubMed allows selected references to be stored online, while further searches are conducted. The results of these further searches can be added to the clipboard, the contents of which can be downloaded and printed when searching is complete. Both PubMed and Ovid offer the facility to view, save, and print results as a text file rather than in hypertext mark up language (HTML) format. Printing in text format saves a considerable amount of paper. Apart from saving and printing text files, you may also wish to save references in a format that can be exported to a reference manager. This is discussed further below.

Although bibliographic databases are immensely powerful, they are not the only source of relevant articles. Many journals are now available electronically, and you may search journals in the area of interest online for relevant material. A number of journals, including the *BMJ* (http://bmj.com/collections) and the *New England Journal of Medicine* (http://content.nejm. org/collections), have electronic archives of previously published papers and reviews, which are organised by subject. Finally, do not neglect the citations in the reference lists of the papers and reviews that you find.

After you have completed your initial literature search and identified relevant references, obtain and read the papers. The abstract of a paper should be an accurate rendition of the contents of the paper, but this is not always the case. A recent study, originally published electronically and described subsequently in *New Scientist*, modelled the way in which errors in citations spread through the literature.[1,2] The study suggested that 78% of citations are "cut and pasted" from a secondary source. The only way to be sure of what a paper says is to read it!

You may find that, no matter how focused you make your bibliographic search, you end up with an unmanageably large number of references. In this case, reading one or two good review articles may provide a gateway to the literature, by explaining the direction of current thought and placing the references you have found in context. If a carefully conducted search yields a large number of references, however, this often indicates that your field of interest is complex and researched widely. It is always wise to seek the advice and support of experts before embarking on new research. If the relevant literature is extensive, expert help is essential.

Managing references

You will find that it does not take long to accumulate a considerable number of paper references. Although storing these in a pile on the corner of your desk keeps them accessible, sooner or later this system will become unmanageable, and your references will start to find their way mysteriously into other piles of paper, on to the floor, and even into the waste bin. Few things are more frustrating than being unable to find a reference that took two weeks to arrive through an interlibrary loan. Devise some simple system for filing and retrieving your papers. I store papers in alphabetical order by the name of the first author. An alternative system involves numbering and storing papers sequentially, and keeping a record of the number in an alphabetical card index or in the database of an electronic reference manager (see below).

Considerably more is involved in managing references than simply keeping track of the paper copies, however. You need to know what the relevance of each reference is, which references you have cited in your manuscript, and the order in which these references come together to form the bibliography of your paper. Traditionally, writers and researchers have done this using a card index system. Each reference is given a numbered index card and the numbers on these cards can be used to indicate citations in a manuscript and to bring together the references for the final bibliography. This system works well, but is labour intensive, and it can become cumbersome when managing a large number of references. The task has been much simplified by the advent of reference management software. A number of different software titles are available; the two most commonly used products are EndNote and Reference Manager – both of which are produced by ISI ResearchSoft.

When you choose which product to use, you should ensure that it is compatible with your word processing software, so that the reference manager and word processor work together to allow you to mark citations in the text and produce a bibliography. You should also be able to import citations from EMBASE, PubMed, and other databases into the reference manager database. These and other tasks are discussed in more detail below. It is often wise to find out which products colleagues use, as they may be able to offer help and support. Local support and licensing arrangements may be available for one or another product.

Reference management software

An electronic reference manager is basically an electronic database that has been adapted to a particular task. It allows you to build up and work with a personal library of references, and this library is therefore at the core of the product. You should be able to view a list of the references that you have stored, sort them by various criteria (such as first author or year of publication), and search them by various criteria. Most reference managers provide a notes section for each reference, in which you can type your own notes as to the relevance and importance of the reference.

One of the great benefits with this software is that references can be imported directly into the reference manager rather than having to be typed in by hand. Most reference managers can recognise and import a variety of different reference formats. The reference or references to be imported are identified in a bibliographic database and are displayed and saved in an importable format. In this format, each field is given a tag that allows it to be identified by other programmes (for example, AU for author and TI for title). The reference manager software is then instructed to import the references from the saved file with the appropriate import format – for example, Medline for references saved from the Medline database. In this way, references may be added to your own database with the minimum of effort and a smaller chance of error than if the references were typed in by hand.

Despite the ease of this process, you need to be aware of some pitfalls. It is easy to import the same reference on a number of different occasions and to end up with several duplicate copies in your reference manager. Check that the authors of each reference are given correctly. If a committee prepared the paper or review, it may be listed in Medline as having no authors. Be aware that the title of the reference given in Medline may carry the suffix "see comments", which refers you to correspondence about the paper. This will have to be removed in your reference manager database before the reference can be exported to your final bibliography. The journal title may be abbreviated, and both the full title and conventional abbreviations may have to be entered into the journals section of your reference manager. Finally, beware the temptation to transfer every reference that you find into your reference manager. Enter only relevant and useful references, because there is no point storing citations that you may never look at again. Databases such as Medline and EMBASE exist to allow you to find such references when you need them.

Referencing your paper

After you have completed your literature search, designed your study, obtained ethical approval, and completed your research, you will finally have reached the stage of writing. In your manuscript, you will need to refer to the works of those who have gone before or perhaps to your own previous research in this field; placing markers in the text that refer the reader to references cited in the reference list or bibliography at the end of your paper. Some of your citations will appear in the introduction to explain why you have undertaken the research, and some may have a place in the methods section to justify and support the methods you have used, but most almost certainly will belong in the discussion, where you seek to explain and interpret your results. You must be selective in your use of references. Most journals limit the number of references that may be appended to a paper. Certainly, no editor will welcome a 1500 word manuscript with 60 references attached. On the other hand, you should cite such material as is necessary to support your work and attempt to produce an inclusive discussion that acknowledges viewpoints other than your own.

It is in the task of referencing a manuscript that reference management software comes into its own. If you use the index card system, each citation has to be marked on the manuscript with an index card number and, when the manuscript is complete, all of the citations have to be collated by hand and a final reference list typed up. An electronic reference manager greatly reduces both the labour involved and the opportunity for error. If the referees request the inclusion of extra references, these can be inserted and the reference list renumbered automatically. If your manuscript, unfortunately, is rejected by one journal and you need to reformat it for submission to another, such reformatting can be done automatically.

The reference manager software and word processor are run in parallel. When the need to cite a reference or references arises, these are identified in the reference manager database, and, with the click of a mouse, unique identifiers for the references are pasted into the text. When the manuscript is complete, the reference manager is instructed to produce a formatted bibliography. The reference manager replaces each citation in the text with an appropriate reference number (Vancouver and related styles) or the name of the first author (Harvard and related styles), and an appropriately formatted reference list is appended to your document. In many programmes, your original file will be overwritten by the new version, so take care to save your original manuscript under a new file name before using the format bibliography command. If you have not kept a version with the citation markers in the text, when the time comes to make corrections to your paper, you may have to go through the manuscript and insert the markers all over again.

Reference formats

Two main formats exist for referencing papers: the Vancouver and the Harvard formats. The former increasingly is preferred for scientific literature. It arose from an informal meeting of a group of editors of medical journals held in Vancouver in 1978. The requirements for manuscripts laid down by the Vancouver group were first published in 1979. The Uniform Requirements for Manuscripts Submitted to Biomedical Journals, as these guidelines have become known, have been through a number of revisions, and journals are now asked to cite a version published in 1997 or later in their instructions to authors.[3,4]

In the Vancouver format, references are numbered consecutively as they appear in the text and are identified by

Arabic numerals in brackets. (Some journals require a different arrangement for review articles, in which the references are arranged alphabetically in the bibliography and numbered accordingly in the text.) In the Harvard system, references are cited in the text by giving the name of the author and the year of the publication in brackets. When a number of references are given together, they should be listed in chronological order separated by semicolons. In the bibliography, the references are listed in alphabetical order by author.

In your manuscript, the reference list at the end of the paper should begin on a new sheet of paper. The fine details of how references should be presented vary from journal to journal, and you should be sure to read the instructions for authors and examine the reference format for the journal to which you plan to submit your manuscript. Many of the reference manager software packages have built into them routines to produce bibliographies for many of the main journals. The usual conventions for the most common forms of citation are given below. Conventions also exist for referencing theses, conference proceedings, and web pages.

Journal article

Surnames and initials of authors. Full title of paper. *Title of journal* Year of publication;**Volume number**:First and last page numbers of article.

Example

Nunn JF, Bergman NA, Coleman AJ. Factors influencing the arterial oxygen tension during anaesthesia with artificial ventilation. *British Journal of Anaesthesia* 1965;**37**:898–914.

Book or monograph

Surname and initials of authors. *Full title of book.* Number of edition. Town of publication: Publisher, Year of publication.

Example

Robinson PN, Hall GM. *How to Survive in Anaesthesia.* 2nd ed. London: BMJ Books, 2002.

Chapter in multi-author book

Chapter author (surnames and initials). Chapter title. Book authors or editors (surnames and initials). *Book title.* Town of publication: Publisher, Year of publication. First and last pages.

Example

Goodman NW. Evidence based medicine: cautions before using. In: Tramèr M, editor. *Evidence Based Resource in Anaesthesia and Analgesia.* London: BMJ Books, 2000. pp 3–22.

Conclusion

Preparation of the references for a paper takes care and organisation. It is not a task that should be neglected; rather the search for relevant references should be the starting point for any research project. Failure to conduct a proper literature search at the outset may lead to embarrassing and potentially serious oversights. It is important not only to obtain the relevant papers, but to read them! When the time to start writing comes, attention to detail in referencing your manuscript and preparing the bibliography is essential. Modern software aids have made the task of managing references much easier, but diligence and care are still necessary. Failure to present an accurate reference list looks sloppy and may encourage the manuscript's assessors to be more critical.

Finally, and perhaps most importantly, finding, reading, and understanding references can be onerous, but do not deny yourself the hidden intellectual pleasures that can come with the task. Discussing the "state of the art" and the formulation of research questions with knowledgeable colleagues may lead you into some fascinating conversations. Furthermore, as time passes and your work progresses, you may come to realise that you have developed quite an authoritative understanding of the state of knowledge in your area of interest. These are quiet, but real, pleasures.

References

1　Simkin MV, Roychowdhury VP. *Read before you cite!* Available from URL: http://www.arxiv.org/abs/cond-mat/0212043.
2　Muir H. Misprinted citations finger scientists who fail to do their homework. *New Scientist* 2002;**176**:12.
3　International Committee of Medical Editors. *Uniform Requirements for Manuscripts submitted to Biomedical Journals.* Available from URL: http://www.icmje.org.
4　International Committee of Medical Editors. *Uniform Requirements for Manuscripts submitted to Biomedical Journals. Ann Intern Med* 1997;**126**: 36–47.

Acknowledgements

I am grateful to Mr Martin Gill, Medical Faculty Team Librarian at the Health Sciences Library of the University of Leeds, for his help and advice in the preparation of this chapter.

8: Electronic submissions

NATALIE DAVIES

The internet has revolutionised our lives completely over the past few years. We can do our grocery shopping, apply for a mortgage, book a holiday, and buy a car from Japan – all in a matter of minutes. We can search for any information we require, and it is ours at the touch of a button. Its time saving properties are unequalled. This revolution has also been transmuted into the medical community. Nearly all of the hundreds of traditional medical journals available have an online version that faithfully mirrors the print journal (and in some cases improves upon it). More and more researchers, academics, and clinicians are turning to the online version, because they know that they can access the information they require much more quickly than searching through piles of paper journals. We are now travelling at an even greater speed down the "information superhighway."

Although revolutionising the lives of consumers, the impact the internet has had on information suppliers, and in this case medical publishers, has been immense. Since the publication of the second edition of this book in 1998, much has changed within medical journal publishing. Maurice Long's chapter, "The future: electronic publishing" foretold some of these changes – notably that "more and more communication between authors, referees, publishers, and readers will be conducted over the net."[1] In the four years since the publication of Long's chapter, this prediction has come to pass for nearly all medical publications.

Electronic submission is not new. The medical community expects the dissemination of research to be speedier than ever before, while still being able to rely on the accuracy of the data. Consequently, authors have demanded that publishers speed up the peer review process and provide quick decisions on papers. This demand has led many journals to utilise the large number of electronic tools available to try and make the peer review process more efficient. Thus, what began as asking for manuscripts to be submitted as electronic copy on disk, progressed to asking for manuscripts to be submitted via email. The next logical step was to use the internet for the submission and review of manuscripts.

Publisher's perspective

At the BMJ Publishing Group, we first began to research the possibility of implementing a web based system in 1999. This was mainly because of the points outlined above, as well as an additional cry from our editors. After evaluating the systems available and testing two of them on two of our journals, we elected to adopt Bench>Press (by HighWire Press) as our system of choice. All the systems available are reasonably similar in construct, allowing authors to use different systems quite painlessly; however, Bench>Press suited our needs better than some of the other systems on the market. An intensive evaluation and implementation programme followed, which was finally completed in October 2002. All BMJ journals now use Bench>Press.

What does web submission mean?

In its simplest form, a web based submission and review system is a database held on a website and accessed via a unique address (URL). This allows authors to access the database from any computer that has access to the internet: whether in the office or home, at a conference centre, or even at a hotel. Authors enter the website, complete a series of fields, upload their manuscript to the database, and *voilà,* the manuscript has been submitted to the journal (see Box 8.1 for detailed author submission guidelines). The old adage of "the manuscript was lost in the post" can no longer be applied. This is not the end of the story, however. Nearly all web based systems in use by publishers offer a fully integrated system that means the *whole* peer review process is also conducted via the website.

Box 8.1 Guidelines for author submission

Please note: terminology and required items may be slightly different depending on the system the journal uses. The terms are usually similar and easily identifiable, however, and the individual journal's "Instructions for authors" should always be read before submission.

1   Access the website via the URL by using a unique user identifier and password
2   Enter the author submission area
3   Choose the "Submit a new manuscript" link
4   Enter the manuscript meta-data. This usually consists of the following basic information: number of authors, type of article, title, manuscript keywords, abstract, cover letter to the editors, author details, suggested reviewers' names, and word count. Most journals ask for extra information, but this is usually explained in the instructions for authors and on the submission pages
5   Enter the number of files you are uploading. This consists of one file for the actual article plus the number of image files associated with the manuscript
6   Search on your computer for your manuscript files and enter the pathway into the appropriate field (for example: C:/My documents/Manuscript title)
7   Follow the system's guidance to "upload" the article to the website
8   The article is converted automatically into a pdf. This is mainly for reviewing purposes and accessibility issues. The pdf file size is smaller than standard word processing and image files, and the software required to view it (Acrobat Reader) is a standard piece of software easily obtained free of charge from the web (http://www.adobe.com)
9   You then have the opportunity to view your submission before it is submitted formally to the journal. This allows you to make sure that what you are submitting is correct and of peer review standard
10 Once approved, the article is then considered to be a formal submission

What happens to the article once it has been submitted?

In the traditional manuscript submission process, authors would submit three or four hard copies of the paper to the editorial office. These would be logged on to a computer, and a copy would be passed to the editor (who is quite often based in a different building, town, or even country) for evaluation. The editor then decided if the manuscript was suitable for the journal and sent his or her decision to the editorial office for action. If the article was considered suitable, it would be posted to suggested reviewers and would then be filed until the reviewers' comments were received. On receipt of the comments, the manuscript again would be posted to the editors for an initial decision. The decision would be made and sent to the editorial office, and a letter posted to the authors. If the initial decision asked the authors to revise their article and resubmit, the manuscript would enter the cycle again. As you can imagine (and may have experienced), this could take an inordinate amount of time. On average, authors could expect to receive an initial decision within 12 weeks, and this does not take into consideration the time taken by those journals that discuss papers with all the editors of the journal at an editorial committee.

Using the web removes many of the above steps. The new internet based systems in place now enable the peer review process to be more streamlined.

- Authors submit their manuscripts online, entering the meta-data traditionally entered by the journal's staff. The manuscript is automatically assigned an identification number, and is entered into the database, from where it is immediately available to editors.
- The editor views the manuscript online and makes an immediate decision or suggests peer reviewers.
- Staff contact the peer reviewers through the web system to ask if they are willing to review the article.
- Reviewers access the reviewers' area of the website and review the paper, submitting their comments via an electronic review form available online.
- Once all comments have been received, the paper and comments are immediately available to the editors, ready for them to make a decision.
- The editor's decision is emailed to the corresponding author.

The above steps show a simplified process, but the benefits the web has brought are obvious. However, authors can gain much more from web submission than purely a reduction in the all-important turnaround times, however.

Benefits of author submission

The benefits to authors are numerous. Not only have the delays inherent in the postal system been made redundant – particularly appreciated by those authors who submit from different countries – but the peer review process has also been made more transparent to authors. Previously, once authors had submitted their manuscript to the journal, they had no way of knowing what was happening until a decision was posted to them by the editors. By accessing the website, authors can now track their paper and see where it is at any given stage; the system allows authors to interact with the process.

Author benefits

1 **Removing the need for "snail mail"**. Manuscripts can no longer be lost or delayed in the post. Authors (or their departments) no longer have the expense of posting three or four hardcopies of the article, which saves on paper, printer cartridges, photographic paper, envelopes, and postage costs.
2 **Approving the article**. Authors can carry out a final check of the paper before submission and correct any mistakes before it is considered. This is important, as some journals do return papers to authors if there is an omission or error, which causes further delays.
3 **Linked references**. Some systems will convert the references of the manuscripts into hyperlinks to Medline or the abstract or full text of the online article (if hosted by HighWire Press). The system also hyperlinks the author's details to all previously published papers. This is an invaluable feature and is much appreciated by editors and reviewers. Please note: the references must be in the *exact* format specified by the journal for optimum linkage. Non-standard journal citations are also difficult to convert.
4. **Supplemental data**. Most web based systems allow authors to upload supplemental data as well as the article

and images. This can be anything from appendices, published articles, questionnaires, and extraneous data.

5 **Interrogation of the system**. Most systems allow authors to view the status of their article as it moves through the peer review process. This provides authors with an easy way to check on the progress of their article, for example, "with editor for decision," "with reviewers awaiting comments," etc.

6 **Contacting the journal**. Email links available throughout the system give authors an easy opportunity to contact journal staff for assistance.

7 **Reviewer's comments available online**. As soon as the editor sends a decision, the reviewer's comments are available online to authors.

8 **Author history**. Authors retain a record on the system of all manuscripts submitted to the journal, including the article itself, the editor's decision letter, and reviewer's comments.

9 **Personal information**. Authors can update their personal details and expertise terms at any time.

10 **Reduced turnaround times**. Perhaps most importantly, turnaround times can be dramatically reduced. At the BMJ Publishing Group, we have seen up to a 50% reduction in time taken to first decision.

Important points to remember

Although most web based systems are reasonably self-explanatory, errors do sometimes occur. This is usually because authors have not properly read the journal's instructions for submission. It is imperative that the instructions are read before submission, as they often contain essential journal requirements as well as guidance on submission. This is particularly important when dealing with images. Most journals and/or web based systems have strict instructions with respect to the format of image files, and it is essential that these are followed. Most systems in use accept the standard graphic formats: .tif, .jpg, .gif, and .eps, and usually there will be no problems with these. If in any doubt, contact the journal's office before submission. Other important points to take note of are:

- *Always* read the instructions for authors before submission and take careful note of journal requirements.
- All systems adopt a strict security system that is based on a user identification (unique email address or other identifier) and password system. This prevents unauthorised access to manuscripts and personal information, and it allows authors to track their manuscript through the process.
- Some systems encrypt passwords for further security and cannot be obtained by journal staff or the software suppliers. In these cases, a "password hint" question and answer system is adopted.
- If the manuscript is accepted, the original word processing and image files (source files) may be requested if the files uploaded to the web based system are not suitable for publication.
- Web based systems are relatively new in a large number of journals and are constantly evolving – mainly in response to authors' comments. Keep that feedback coming in!
- If in any doubt, contact the staff of the editorial office, who will always be happy to help.

The future

The adoption of an electronic submission and peer review system may well help reduce the time from submission to decision; however, we are still living in a largely print based world. The time from acceptance to publication can still be lengthy, and many journals have to limit the length of articles because of page restrictions. Many publishers are now starting to scrutinise this end of the process and to utilise the myriad benefits of the internet to provide improvements. Such innovations include:

- publish ahead of print: articles are published online before publication in the print journal – in some cases, this can be some months in advance
- publish online instead of in print
- e-letters: authors can post immediate responses to published articles online
- "short" versions of the paper in print, with a longer, more detailed version online.

Many journals are also beginning to offer added "web" benefits, including: movies, extra images, data supplements, presentations, coming events, email alerts, cite track (this allows the author to track topics and authors in any of the participating journals), journal announcements, enhanced searching and display across topics and journals, course material, interactive educational material, and the facility to download articles to a personal digital assistant (PDA).

From the innovations listed above, the future may already seem to be here. Not so. New technologies are being developed quicker than ever. Medicine is constantly evolving. Our authors' and readers' needs change. All of the innovations already in place are there in response to our authors' requirements. As such, everyone involved in the medical community – authors, reviewers, editors, readers, as well as publishers – can expect an exciting few years ahead!

Reference

1   Long M. The Future: Electronic Publishing. In: Hall GM, ed. *How to Write a Paper*. Second edition. London: BMJ Publishing Group, 1998:132–7.

9: How to write a letter

MICHAEL DOHERTY

General considerations

When you think of submitting a letter to a journal, first consider the following basic questions:

- What is the purpose of your letter?
- Is a letter format appropriate for this particular journal?
- Does what you want to say justify a communication?

The purpose of a letter varies between journals (Box 9.1). Most letters are comments in response to a previous publication, although brief communications that do not justify an extended or concise report are sometimes appropriate as letters. It is always wise to read the "Instructions for authors" and to examine the correspondence section of recent issues of the journal to gain a feel for the style and scope of successful (that is, published!) letters. Because the amount of information provided in a letter is necessarily limited, rarely is there justification for a long list of authors. Always question whether the information you wish to convey truly justifies publication – minor comments or observations are unlikely to be accepted.

If the purpose and content of your communication seem appropriate as a letter, two other major considerations are its length and the style of presentation. With respect to length, always be brief. Editors like concise communications. They would rather publish 10 short letters on 10 different topics than two lengthy ones on only two topics. Think how you react as a reader – messages are always more effective if put succinctly. Some journals impose firm restrictions on word count, number of references, and use of accompanying tables or figures, and these restrictions will be outlined in their

---

> **Box 9.1 The purpose of a letter**
>
> **Usual**
>
> - Comment (positive or negative) in response to a previous publication
> - Concise communication of clinical or investigative data
> - Communication of case report(s)
>
> **Less common**
>
> - General medical or political comment (for example, "guild issues")
> - Comment concerning the nature or format of the journal
> - Advertisement of interest to collaborate or to gain access to patients or study material

instructions to authors. Even if not overtly stated, however, all editors favour a "Raymond Chandler" over a "Charles Dickens". For example, compare the following two introductory paragraphs to the same letter.

Sir,

I feel I must put pen to paper with respect to the recent communication by Dr Peter Jones and colleagues in your August issue,[1] to draw the attention of your readers to possible misinterpretation of the data that they present. Although these excellent workers have an internationally renowned track record in the field of complement activation (not only in rheumatoid arthritis but in other inflammatory diseases as well), in this present study, they seem to have omitted to properly control for the varying degrees of inflammation in the knee joints of the patients that they aspirated – not only those with rheumatoid arthritis but also those with osteoarthritis. Such inflammation of the knee joint could have been assessed readily either by local examination and scoring of features such as temperature increase, effusion, synovial thickening, anterior joint line tenderness, duration of early morning stiffness, and the duration of inactivity stiffness, with addition of the different scores to a single numerical value (that is, the system devised and tested by Robin Cooke and colleagues in Alberta[2]) and/or by simultaneous measurement and comparison to levels of other markers of inflammation, for example, the synovial fluid total white cell and differential (particularly polymorphonuclear cell) count or local synovial fluid levels of various arachidonic acid products such as prostaglandins or leukotrienes ...

(Dr C Dickens)

Sir,
In their study of synovial fluid complement activation Jones *et al*[1] made no assessment of the inflammatory state of aspirated knees. Such assessment could have been attempted using the summated six-point clinical scoring system of Cooke *et al*[2] or by estimation of alternative indicators of inflammation (for example, cell counts, prostaglandins, or leukotrienes).
(Dr R Chandler)

Both convey the same message. The second is more "punchy", however, and gets straight to the point by omitting unnecessary description and detail. As with any scientific writing, keep sentences short. Make each of your points separately. Reference short statements rather than provide extended summaries of previous work.

Etiquette and style for letters in response to an article

A letter is the accepted format for comment relating to a previous publication in the same journal. Occasionally it may relate to a publication in another journal. Note that letters are always directed to the editor, never to the initial author. The editor in this situation is an impartial intermediary between authors, particularly those in potential conflict.

The usual purpose of a responding letter is to offer support or criticism (most commonly criticism) of the rationale, method, analysis, or conclusion of the previous study. If this is the case, make specific, reasoned criticisms or provide additional pertinent data to be considered in the topic under consideration (Box 9.2). Do not reiterate arguments already fully covered or referenced in the provoking publication. Your letter should raise new points that were not addressed adequately or should provide additional information that supports or refutes the contentions of the other authors. However prestigious you may think yourself, merely offering your personal dissent or approval is not enough. You should use the letter to argue a reasoned perspective. It should not be a vehicle for biased opinion. Always be specific. General comments unsubstantiated by reasoned argument ("I think this a great publication" or "I think it is rubbish") are unacceptable.

> **Box 9.2 Guidelines for a letter in response to an article**
>
> - Be courteous and interested – not rude or dismissive
> - Make specific rather than general comments
> - Give reasoned argument, not biased opinion
> - Do not repeat aspects already covered in the original article
> - Introduce a different perspective or additional data to the topic
> - Attempt to make only one or a very few specific points
> - Be concise

If you are offering criticism, always be professional and courteous – never rude, arrogant, or condescending. Apart from common decency to fellow investigators, politeness in correspondence will serve to enhance and safeguard whatever reputation you have. This is the same golden rule that applies to question time at oral presentations. No one likes a rude critic, even (or more especially) one who is right. A polite, understated question or comment inevitably has more critical impact than arrogant dismissal. For example, compare the following two styles of presentation. Both letters make the same points.

Sir,

I was greatly surprised that the paper on synovial fluid complement breakdown products (C3dg) by Jones et al[1] managed to get into your journal. Firstly, Jones et al[1] obviously forgot to control for the inflammatory state of the knees that they aspirated, even though our group previously has drawn attention to the importance of this in any study of synovial fluid.[2] Secondly, they made no attempt to determine levels of C3dg in synovial fluid from normal knees. Since they only compared findings between knees of patients with either rheumatoid or pyrophosphate arthritis, it is hardly surprising that they jump to the wrong conclusion in stating that complement activation is not a prominent feature of pyrophosphate arthropathy. Thirdly, they only reported crude C3dg concentrations, with no correction for synovial fluid native C3 levels. If these investigators had only taken the time to read the existing literature, they would have realised that we previously have shown that such correction is of paramount importance for correct interpretation of C3dg data. That such a majorly flawed paper, which does not even reference our seminal work,[2] should be published at all – let alone as an extended paper – must seriously question the effectiveness of the peer review system that you operate.

A Pratt

Sir,

I was interested in the study of synovial fluid breakdown products (C3dg) by Jones *et al*,[1] in which they conclude, contrary to our previous report,[2] that complement activation is not a feature of chronic pyrophosphate arthropathy. Such discordance most likely relates to differences in clinical characterisation and expression of C3dg levels rather than to estimation of C3dg itself. Unlike Jones *et al*, we assessed and controlled for the inflammatory state of aspirated knees, included normal knees as a control group, and corrected for native C3 concentrations (expressed as a ratio C3dg/C3), as well as reporting C3dg concentrations. By employing these methods, we were able to demonstrate complement activation in clinically inflamed, but not quiescent, pyrophosphate arthritis knees. Such activation was less marked quantitatively than that observed in active rheumatoid knees. We would suggest that clinical assessment of inflammatory state, inclusion of normal knee controls, and correction for native C3 levels be considered in future studies of synovial fluid.

A Diplomat

Remember that the original authors will usually be invited to respond to your criticisms. It is much easier to respond to a rude than a polite letter, and even potentially damning points that you raise may get lost in the "noise" of confrontation. For example, Dr Jones would be able to centre his reply to Dr Pratt's letter on the defence of the peer review system. He would be hard pressed, however, to sidestep the same specific criticisms levelled by Dr Diplomat. Furthermore, the original authors have the last word, and if your criticisms are misplaced (it happens!) you may not be given the opportunity to rescind before publication. You may then find yourself publicly ridiculed, appearing as a rude ignoramus rather than an interested and inquiring intellectual. For example:

Sir,

We are grateful to Dr Pratt for his comments. We in fact had carefully considered all the points he raises. Because all knees included in our study were clinically inflamed, the question of correcting for differing degrees of inflammation does not arise. We also considered aspiration of normal knees, but this was not approved by our research ethics committee. We included estimation of native C3 and expression of C3dg/C3 in our original manuscript. This made no difference to the results and, because the main thrust of our paper dealt with the method – not the demonstration – of C3 activation in rheumatoid knees (with original data on C4d and factor B activation), we were asked to delete these data by the expert reviewers. We of course were aware of the study by Dr Pratt and colleagues, but we were limited in the number of references we could include. We referred therefore to the first report of synovial fluid C3dg in normal, rheumatoid, and pyrophosphate arthritis knees by Earnest *et al*,[1] which predated that of Pratt *et al* by six years.

Other forms of letter

In many journals, the correspondence section is an appropriate site for short reports that have a simple message but do not necessitate a full paper. This is particularly true if a study uses standard techniques that are readily referenced and require no detailed explanation.

Studies

Presentation of a study as a letter is rather similar to writing an extended abstract (Box 9.3). Normally there should be three clear divisions: an introduction relating the rationale and objectives of the study; a section stating the methods, analysis, and results; and, finally, a conclusion. The conclusion should assess the validity and importance of the findings in the context of other work, highlight the caveats and strengths of the study, and indicate the direction of future related research. Unlike concise or extended reports, section headings are not enforced, and an abstract is unnecessary. Nevertheless, subheadings may be used to good effect and often assist the clarity of presentation.

Although often considered a "second-rate" way of reporting data, a letter format is quite appropriate for brief reports and can still be prestigious, especially in high impact journals. If you are presenting original data in a letter, carefully consider whether this will compromise subsequent publication of the same data in a more extended form. Remember that letters can be referenced and that "redundant" or duplicate publications must be avoided.

> **Box 9.3 Presentation of a concise report as a letter**
>
> Introduce the topic
> - Briefly explain rationale and objectives of study
>
> Present methods and results
> - Reference methods as much as possible
> - Include only essential data
> - If possible present data in a table and/or figure
>
> Present conclusions
> - Emphasise only one or a few major conclusions
> - Avoid extrapolating too far from data
> - Highlight caveats and strengths of the study
> - Suggest future studies that are still required in this area
>
> Avoid repetition of data or conclusions
> Be concise

Case reports

Case reports are often presented as letters. They are particularly suitable for single cases that do not justify a full or concise report. Some journals have no specific slot for case reports and publish all cases as letters. Most editors only publish cases that give novel insight into pathogenesis, diagnosis, or management. To report the sixth case of concurrence of two diseases in the same patient is of no scientific interest – only a formal study, not further case reports, can answer whether this is chance concurrence or a true association that may give clues relating to pathogenesis of either disease. As with short reports, cases are best divided into a brief introduction, a description of the case itself, and then a discussion of its interest, with no section headings. Be particularly careful not to repeat the same information by summarising the case at the beginning and the end. This is a common and easy mistake.

General or political comment

General or political comment occurs mainly in major weekly journals or in specialist journals that are the official outlet of learned societies. In this situation, humorous comments may be permitted. Humour is always risky, however – especially for an international audience with diverse perspectives on what, if anything, is funny. Letters may be used to advertise an interest in particular cases or investigational material for research purposes or a service on offer (for example, DNA repository). Such advertisements should be very brief and are more usually found in a notes or news section.

10: How to prepare an abstract for a scientific meeting

ROBERT N ALLAN

Introduction

It is, of course, preposterous that anyone should insist that your work, which is at the forefront of scientific development and has consumed your life for the last 12 months, should be reduced to an abstract box. Pause, recover your equilibrium, and muster a little sympathy for the organisers of the meeting at which you wish to present your original work.

The scientific programme will have been planned several years in advance. The lectures and symposia will have been agreed, the national and international speakers invited, and the venue selected. In addition, the programme will include a limited number of spaces for presentation of abstracts, either as oral communications or posters.

Selection of abstracts

As the number of abstracts submitted usually exceeds the number that can be included, some sort of selection procedure must be used. A panel of reviewers, each an expert in their own field, is asked to assess each abstract. Each reviewer has a large number of abstracts to assess, so the time allocated to your own precious abstract may well be short. Furthermore, the secretariat organising the meeting will know that authors often ignore instructions and submit abstracts which are over length, illegible, incomplete, and late. They will be determined on this occasion only to consider abstracts that conform to the published guidelines. Be warned!

Online submission of abstracts

Online submission is now common for abstracts. The website of the society organising the meeting will include detailed information, and many meetings have a site dedicated to preparation of abstracts. For example, the British Society of Gastroenterology's home page (http://www.bsg.org.uk) provides clear instructions, with direct access to the abstract submission website (http://www.bsgabstracts.org.uk).

Guidelines for online submission

Specific guidelines must be followed – type only within the specified area and include the title, list of authors, institution, and address. Do not modify the page setup with respect to dimensions or font (print) size. You must declare originality or previous publication.

Snail mail submissions

Guidelines

The instructions for postal submissions may look (and usually are!) tedious, but they are designed to ensure high quality reproduction of your work. Abstracts are now rarely edited and typeset – an approach that produced well presented abstracts, regardless of the quality of the original. For speed and efficiency, abstracts may be photographed and reproduced exactly as they first appear (camera ready abstracts). The abstract therefore must be typed within the prescribed area. An appropriate size typeface and a high quality laser printer should be used to ensure good reproduction. Direct reproduction of the camera ready abstract will mean that any errors in spelling, grammar, or scientific fact will be reproduced exactly as you typed them, so take care. Vain hopes that the photographic process might in some way enhance your abstract must be abandoned.

Send the appropriate number of copies. Anonymous copies – without the names of the author and the institution where the work was carried out – are often requested to ensure that the marking system is independent and fair. Make a careful note of the deadline – preparation of abstracts always takes longer than expected. Late entries or those not conforming to the guidelines may be rejected out of hand, without evaluation.

The abstract form commonly includes a number of subject categories. Identify the most appropriate category for your work to ensure that the selected reviewer is an expert in your field. Mark whether the abstract will be presented as a poster or oral presentation. You must declare that the abstract is completely original or to submit details if the abstract has been submitted to another meeting or for publication. Full information must be provided.

Preparation of the abstract

The abstract should be prepared with a number of headings – even though the headings themselves may eventually be deleted from the final text.

Title

The title is a concise summary of the abstract and must demonstrate that the work is important, relevant, and innovative. Define the key features of your work and link them together until the title effectively conveys that message.

Authors

Include authors who really have contributed to the work. It is assumed, if the abstract is accepted, that the first author will present the work. The author who presents the work often has to be identified. The name and address of the institution at which the work was carried out is included, with an email address where the authors can be reached if problems arise. For example, your abstract may be selected for a plenary session, and the organisers will need to confirm that the presenter speaks fluent English and that the work is sufficiently important for such a session.

Background

Start with a sentence or two that summarises previous work relevant to the presentation. Highlight any controversies that your work has helped to resolve.

Aims

What is the point of the study? What is the hypothesis that is being addressed? How is your work different from previous work? Is it useful, exciting, and worthwhile? Does it make a new and significant contribution? To encapsulate these ideas in a sentence or two takes practice.

Patients

If patients were studied, how were they selected? Did they give informed consent? Was the selection of patients random? Why were patients excluded? Was ethical committee approval obtained?

Methods

The techniques employed must be summarised and novel methods described in greater detail. Minimise the use of abbreviations, which may confuse the reader and assessor. Note the methods used to test for statistical significance.

Results

Data about patients should be described first, including the numbers studied, sex, age, distribution, and duration of follow up. The key results should then be summarised, usually in four or five sentences that identify the positive features; ensure that any claims can be substantiated. Highlight new developments.

Discussion

What has the work added to the existing body of knowledge? In what way are these new findings important? Could the findings have occurred by chance or are they statistically significant?

Conclusions

Why is the work important? How might the work be developed further?

From draft to final version

The draft abstract is now complete. It will be hopelessly over length. To produce this information in an abstract of less than 200 words is a real challenge. Delete any duplicated, superfluous, or irrelevant information. Can the same idea be conveyed in fewer words? If the abstract is still over length, what are the most important results? Can some points be omitted and presented separately at the meeting?

It will take time and many drafts to produce the final version. Start early and plan to complete and submit the abstract well before the deadline. The abstract must summarise the work, but do not forget that it must excite the reviewer in that "brief moment of time" when your abstract is assessed.

Reread the guidelines and ensure that you, your word processor, and secretary have conformed completely with the instructions. Photocopy the original abstract form and ensure that the draft abstract can be laid out effectively within the space available. Circulate the draft abstract to your colleagues and obtain their approval before submission.

Final preparation

The abstract can now be completed and the appropriate number of named and anonymous copies prepared. Do not duplicate submissions – two or more abstracts that describe similar results from the same study are both likely to be rejected. Include an email address to learn the outcome of the assessor's evaluation.

Outcome

In due course, you will hear the outcome of the assessment and experience the joy of acceptance or the depression of rejection. Few abstracts are outstanding, and few are awful. The marks for most abstracts hover around the mean and abstracts are either just accepted or just rejected. Temper the joy of acceptance with modesty. The depression of rejection can be minimised by knowing that the abstract was only just rejected.

Presenting the data

The accepted abstract has to be converted into an oral presentation or a poster – another exciting challenge. Submission of an abstract implies that one of the authors will present the paper or poster in person at the meeting. Late withdrawal of an abstract gives the individual and their unit a bad name.

Conclusion

An abstract that effectively summarises your work clearly and concisely with an apparently effortless presentation can be achieved only with meticulous preparation. In doing so, however, you will share in the excitement of contributing at the forefront of new scientific developments.

11: How to write a case report

JAW WILDSMITH

Case reporting is arguably the oldest and most basic form of communication in medicine. The verbal presentation and explanation of a case history is a skill acquired early in undergraduate training and one that most clinicians use throughout their careers. Much the same ability is required to make a written presentation: the positive features have to be detailed in a sequential and logical fashion, together with "negative" material that is directly relevant. A case report is, for many clinicians, the first entry into print and, because the basic method is familiar, it is a useful exercise in learning how to write.

That point made, it is important to remember that all the rules that apply to other forms of medical writing apply equally to case reports. Clear, unambiguous English should be used to present the material, so that the reader has a clear understanding of:

- what happened to the patient
- the time course of these events
- why management followed the lines that it did.

The key feature of a good case report is that it should help the reader to recognise and deal with a similar problem should one ever present itself.

In preparing a case report, the writer should be asking three questions:

- What am I going to report?
- How should I report it?
- In which journal am I aiming to publish the report?

What to report

Most doctors occasionally come across a patient whose condition might merit production of a case report. The key is both to observe and to think about clinical practice. In today's circumstances, only a very lucky doctor will describe a totally original condition, but many rare or unusual patients may merit description. Rarity is not in itself, however, cause for publication. The case must be special and have a "message" for the reader. It could be to raise awareness of the condition so that the diagnosis may be made more readily in the future, or the report might indicate how one line of treatment was more suitable and effective than another. What such case reports do – to draw a legal parallel – is establish "case law" for relatively rare disease states.

The second group of patients who may be worth reporting comprises those with unusual, perhaps even unknown, conjunctions of conditions, which may have opposing priorities in their managements. A variation on this theme is the patient who presents with a rare or unusual complication of a disease or therapeutic procedure. Again, although it is important to indicate what message there is in *this* patient's case for those who read about it, almost as important as the message is that the case should be interesting to read about. Clearly, skill as an author is going to influence readability, but no amount of writing skill is going to make an uneventful case interesting.

You would do well to remember from the beginning that the first reader of the report will be the editor. Although some editors are totally averse, many feel that case reports help attract readers by making their journals seem a little more relevant to "ordinary" clinicians who feel that the more scientific contributions do not interest them immediately. Most editors whose journals include case reports receive many more than they have space to publish, so the writer must ensure that the report is unusual, interesting, and readable, to give it the best chance of being accepted.

Assess the potential response

When deciding whether your case meets the above criteria, it would be useful for you to consider how others might respond to the details. A review of the literature may indicate that your case is rare or unusual, but a literature review is time consuming and expensive. It may be more helpful initially to describe the patient to two or three colleagues of varying seniority to see their responses. Thereafter, verbal presentation at a departmental meeting will help refine your product. What is rare in one hospital, however, may be commonplace in another because of differences in referral patterns. What seems unusual to you may be relatively routine elsewhere, and sooner or later you will need to do a literature search. It is also necessary to ensure that the motive for publishing the case is not self-aggrandisement. It is the patient who should be interesting, not the author's skill in diagnosis or management. All of these issues are particularly relevant if you are considering the publication of a series of similar patients, because only rarely will this provide genuinely new insights into the incidence, characteristics, or other aspects of the condition.

Many modern case reports describe complications, and these can produce a range of responses. Ideally, such a report should make the reader grateful that he or she was not involved but intrigued at what happened. It should indicate also how the problem could be avoided in the future. It is but a small step, however, from here to the reader feeling that somebody (and sometimes everybody) involved in the management of the patient made a complete mess of it. The report thus may extend a publication list but do nothing for professional reputation! Conversely, in these audit conscious days, we are encouraged more to "own up" when things go wrong, and such reports have merit if the message is clear to others. The *BMJ* encourages this under the general heading of "Lesson of the Week." A variation on this theme is the publication of a series of patients in whom there have been similar complications. The strength of the message is greater than if only a single case had been described, but that message must be applicable to *current* practice. Unfortunately, most such series accrue to doctors involved with patients seeking redress for their problems through the courts, and the length of the medicolegal process means that it may be many years before the details can be published.

How to report

After you have established that your case is of interest to others, you need to ensure that the material is presented in a fashion that will make others share your interest. It is probably wise to start by writing down (for your initial verbal presentation) the details of the case, then to develop the discussion, and finally to add the other components. This is not the way in which the reader will encounter the report, however, and the overall sequence must be kept in mind throughout.

Title

Most journal readers decide which papers they are going to read by skimming the titles. If the title of a case report is too full, the reader may feel it has said all there is to know. Ideally the title should be short, descriptive, and eye catching.

Authorship

Establishing authorship is an increasing problem in medical publication, and this applies particularly to case reports. Only one person should actually write the paper, with the other authors restricted to those who had a significant input to the management of those aspects that were unusual. A case report written by two or three individuals may be reasonable, therefore, but it is difficult to see any justification for a list of five or six authors to describe the management of one patient. This smacks of ego "massaging" in the interests of the future advancement of the first named author.

Introduction

There is a tendency to write a short history of the condition when introducing a case report, but this is either unnecessary material or it should be put in the discussion. Certainly, the introduction may be used to place the case in context or indicate its relevance, but often there is no need to have an opening section at all. The report may begin simply with the case description.

Case description

When you write the core part of the paper, it is essential that you keep to the basic rules of clinical practice. The details will vary a little according to the specialty, but the report should be chronological and detail the presenting history, examination findings, and investigation results before going on to describe the patient's progress. The description should be complete, but the real skill is to accentuate the positive features without obscuring them in a mass of negative and mostly irrelevant findings. Consider what questions of fact a colleague might ask (this is one reason for an initial verbal presentation) and ensure that the answers are presented clearly within the report. Illustrations can be particularly helpful, and in some circumstances they are essential. A photograph of the patient or the equipment used, line diagrams of operative procedures, graphs of physiological measurements, and summary tables of events can all, when used appropriately, add much to the reader's understanding.

Never forget that it is a patient who is being described – not a case – and that confidentiality must be absolute. Age, occupation, and geographical location might be all that a determined journalist needs to identify the patient, yet such information can be essential to the report. Similarly, blanking over the eyes may be enough to obscure identity only if the reader does not know the individual. Increasingly, it may be wise to obtain written consent from the patient at an early stage in the preparation of the report, particularly if photographic material is to be used. Many journals now insist on this.

Discussion

When you are preparing a report of an unusual condition, it will often be tempting to expand the paper and produce a review of the literature – particularly if a great deal of work has been put into gathering all the published information on the condition. This is a temptation that should be resisted (by editors as well as authors). If a review is merited, it should be written in an entirely separate exercise by a much more experienced author than is usual for a case report.

The main purpose of the discussion is to explain how and why decisions were made and what lesson is to be learnt from *this* experience. Some reference to other cases may be required, but, again, the tendency to produce a review must be resisted. The aim should be to refine and define the message for the reader. A good case report will make it quite clear how such a patient would be managed in the future.

References

As indicated above, reference to the work of others should be made only where needed to make a clear point. If a standard textbook has indicated that one line of treatment should have been followed, then it should be quoted. Reports by others should be mentioned only where they actively support (or contradict) the particular experience and conclusion.

No matter how exhaustive your search of the literature has been, something may have been missed out. Only a very brave, or perhaps foolhardy, author claims absolute priority in the description of some clinical phenomenon.

Acknowledgements

Acknowledgement of the assistance and support of others is almost as difficult an area as the decision about who should be included as authors of a case report. The key question is whether the patient would have been managed or the paper written without the assistance of that specific individual. A particular problem is deciding whether it is necessary to thank the consultant or other individual clinically responsible for the patient for permission to publish details. With the modern tendency to seek permission from the patient, this rather old fashioned practice is dying out.

Where to publish

A provisional decision about which journal the report will be submitted to should be made before starting to write. The next stage must be to read the guidelines to contributors. Journals vary in style and it is helpful to try and picture how the report will appear in print while you are preparing it. The author should always aim for a peer reviewed journal and one that he or she already reads regularly. Familiarity with the journal will provide a better idea of what the editor, and thus the readers, find interesting, and this will help with the whole process of preparation.

Thereafter, your decision will be between submitting to a general, specialist, or even subspecialty journal. The choice

---

Box 11.1 Guidelines for a case report

- The report should detail:

  - What happened to the patient
  - The time course of events
  - Why the particular management was chosen

- An opening section may not be needed. Begin with the case description if possible
- Positive features should be accentuated and irrelevant details avoided
- A photograph or other illustration may be useful
- Confidentiality must be absolute
- The discussion should be useful and not overlong
- Reference other work only when necessary to make a specific point
- Cases that really merit publication always have an educational message

---

will depend on the rarity of the case and its specific features. Keep in mind the basic reason for writing a case report: namely, that it should have a message for the reader. Decide what the message is, consider who the message is aimed at, and then select a journal whose readership will include the target audience.

The final stages of preparation

Once the first draft is written, you should put it away for a week or two, then refine it and revise it several times. Reading the report aloud – first in private and later to one or two others who have not heard the case before – is an invaluable exercise. This will help improve the clarity of the report and its English, as well as bringing out any inconsistencies of fact or interpretation. The text should be checked and rechecked for errors in spelling, punctuation, and adherence to the journal's instructions on style. Finally, the requisite number of clear copies, correctly paginated, should be sent with a polite covering letter to the editor – accompanied by a silent prayer that the next issue of that journal does not contain a description of an identical patient!

12: How to write a review

IAN FORGACS

Review articles are in a state of somewhat uncontrolled proliferation. Both general and specialist journals have grown to love them, and considerable growth has been seen in the number of publications devoted just to publishing reviews. Yet, unquestionably the task of writing a review article has become a whole lot tougher in recent years. The days are surely numbered when it is acceptable for an editor to offer the numero uno top banana in the field a modest (and they always are modest) honorarium in exchange for a few thousand words on the great man's reflections on the contentious areas in his particular specialty. For areas in which a wealth of valuable data exists, the personal perspective has gone out of fashion, and in has come the systematic review, as the careful weighing of evidence has surpassed the *ex cathedra* overview.

Of course, whole areas where there is a lack or, at very least, a paucity of evidence remain, and the more traditional or narrative review retains its place for these. Even here, however, it has become necessary for authors of such reviews to declare the sources on which their opinions are founded.

Who needs review articles?

Journal editors like reviews. The thorough, authoritative review is likely to be widely read and highly cited, and this may increase the journal's impact factor (a measure of a journal's success). In addition, many journals that depend heavily on publishing original science face competition from the internet and have been looking for ways to attract readers. Expansion of a paper journal's educational role is seen as one route to ensure a viable future. Readers also turn to a review article as they feel that, like a morning jog or cold shower, the effort involved might actually improve them. Market research suggests that, although readers may skim original material, they tend to make the effort to read topical reviews in the unequal struggle to keep up to date. In other words, reading reviews is good for you. Many specialties have journals that consist of little more than a collection of reviews; these usually are worthy but dull. Indeed, many review articles often are quite tedious, although they don't have to be. It is absolutely essential that those who write reviews transmit the enthusiasm that carries them through the working day. This chapter aims to help you write an article that might actually be read by someone other than the author, the editor, and the proofreader.

Who should write a review?

Editors will usually try to persuade someone right at the cutting edge of a particular field to provide the article. In general, the further the author is from the frontier of knowledge in that particular area, the less well informed is the review. From time to time, journals receive unsolicited review articles for consideration. In many instances, such pieces read uncannily like the introductory chapter of a thesis or dissertation – and are invariably only too lightly disguised! Editors should spare their readers these unauthoritative and dreary offerings. If you experience the desire to write a review for a particular journal, first go for a brisk walk in a nearby park. If you still feel the need to share your thoughts on a specific topic with the world at large, do make polite enquiry of the editor as to how such a piece might be received before putting pen to paper.

Many journal editors report increasing difficulty in recruiting authors to write reviews. A law of inverse proportionality exists: both the likelihood of an author accepting a commission and the number of its eventual readers are inversely proportional to the required length of article. Clearly, it is in everyone's interest to keep article length under control. There is no shortage of eminent folk only too willing to put together a commentary or leading article of up to 1500 words, but it is becoming harder and harder to persuade the great and the good to write reviews. The mutually acceptable answer may be to accept co-authorship

> **Box 12.1**
>
> - A meta-analysis is research in which data from separate studies that address a similar research question are combined quantitatively and then analysed statistically.
> - A systematic review is a review article based on data from original research studies that have been selected in an objective and rigorous manner following a defined method.

between the desired star name and a less well established colleague. Clearly the junior partner(s) will do most of the real work, but an editor can reasonably expect that the finished product represents real collaborative effort.

Writing a systematic review

Unfortunately, some confusion exists over the meanings of the terms "meta-analysis". and "systematic review" (see Box 12.1). Meta-analysis is, in effect, a piece of research that combines evidence from a number of separate studies in a quantitative manner. By careful use of original data, meta-analysis has the potential to provide a more precise effect of a particular intervention than can be gained from the results of individual clinical trials.

Although meta-analyses can be considered to be original statistical research, systematic reviews involve the balanced assessment of original research studies. Conclusions are drawn not from mathematical summation, but from an objective review of relevant studies that have to meet acceptable criteria of quality. Although the meta-analyst and systematic reviewer both need to apply rigorous criteria when selecting the appropriate material for their endeavours, the meta-analyst goes for a mathematical synthesis, while the reviewer settles for a balanced yet critical summary. The main advantage of being systematic is that the personal views and prejudices of the author are suppressed by the weight of objectivity. In modern jargon, being systematic means being evidence based, and such reviews have become increasingly important in a world in which clinical effectiveness is translated into clinical governance.

Box 12.2 Obtaining the data

- Search through computerised databases – Medline, EMBASE, Cochrane Library
- Use personal knowledge of the relevant literature
- Check the reference lists of papers
- Hand search the key journals

Finding the data (Box 12.2)

Computerised searches are very helpful, but almost invariably they are not complete. Access to large databases such as Medline, EMBASE, and the Cochrane Library is readily available in all libraries, in most clinical and academic departments, and, increasingly, in the homes of internet-connected medical authors. Searching does take some practice but, with a combination of luck, tact, and charm, your local librarian can be a helpful tutor in search techniques. You may really need guidance on how to focus on your specific area of interest if your initial search reveals several thousand articles!

Nevertheless, even the best databases are incomplete. Personal knowledge of the field (a *sine qua non* for a reviewer) nearly always throws up articles not revealed by computer searches. A check of the references of the various papers is helpful and can be supplemented by a manual search of the title pages of the key journals in the field. Publication bias (the tendency for trials with negative results never to see the printed page) means that a fully systematic search might involve a direct approach to authors to ask if they have (or know of) unpublished data. Such thoroughness would be regarded by most editors as a counsel of perfection, but it would be appropriate to ensure that your review marshalled the data as comprehensively as possible. In particular, it is necessary to emphasise the results of studies that are well designed, and this is especially important in assimilating data from clinical trials. It can be very helpful to tabulate the outcome of a series of studies, and the merit of such a table is strengthened by giving some indication of those studies that report the results of good quality, randomised, double blind, controlled clinical trials.

A good review should do more than just present the data, and readers expect a reward for the time they spend reading your prose – in the form of some sort of conclusion. Remember that readers who are running out of time or stamina really appreciate a clear summary, which most usually should be offered in the form of bullet points.

Writing a narrative review

The systematic review lends itself to specific topics in which there exists a body of data concerning particular intervention(s) in clinical practice – for example, the role of a specific pharmacological intervention in the management of acute myocardial infarction or the value of interventional endoscopy in upper gastrointestinal haemorrhage. Yet in many areas, being systematic just is not possible; this may be because no comparative data are available or because the whole subject area is not one that can be evaluated by such methods. One cannot be systematic in a review article on the molecular genetics of breast cancer. It is important, however, for the reviewer to amass the key material so as to avoid personal bias in favour of a particular viewpoint. The most serious crime that a review author can commit is to be partial.

Whether being systematic or narrative, the most time consuming aspect of putting together a review article is collecting the source material. If this has not taken up nine tenths of your total time on the whole project, you are exceptionally well organised, lucky, or insufficiently prepared.

Constructing the article (Box 12.3)

An eye catching title can be a good start, but you should avoid flippancy. A review article on recent progress in extracorporeal shockwave lithotripsy in cholelithiasis can be cheered up by such a title as "Shock news for gallstones". The opening paragraphs are the most crucial in the whole piece. By the end of the first page, you should have explained to the readers exactly what your piece is about, convinced them that the article is worth reading, and demonstrated that what you have to say is informed, authoritative, and interesting. Many otherwise able reviews are condemned to be read by no more folk than can gather together in a phone box because of verbal tedium.

Box 12.3 Constructing the review

- Effective title
- Clear introduction

    - What the article is about
    - Say why it is worth reading
    - Make it clear you are informed and interesting

- Statement of how the data were selected
- Presentation of the data
- Clear conclusions

Often the first sentences of any article are the hardest to write and, once a few hundred words have appeared on screen, writing all seems to become rather easier. Although I do not belong to the school of endless drafts and redrafts, few final versions of medical articles have not benefited from radical excision from earliest drafts of the first couple of hundred words – they usually say little and mean even less. My editorial red pen is never wielded more energetically than when the author has failed to follow this guideline.

Medical journals are increasingly formulating quite strict guidelines for authors of reviews. Although there is some danger that, in itself, a standard format can be mind numbingly dull, at least it ensures that the article meets the minimum criteria set by the journal. It is becoming standard practice for the author to be required to state, quite early on in the review, how he selected the information on which the review was based. Although journals, thankfully, are still a long way from adopting the view that all reviews must be systematic, they do expect that the author will reveal how the material was selected. A journal's reputation can be dented seriously by a maverick author who bases a piece on a highly selective perspective of the literature. Potential readers should be able to judge quite rapidly what sort of effort the author has made in marshalling the facts before they themselves make the effort to plough through the prose.

The body of data should be presented in a form in which justice is done to its level of complexity but notice is also taken of the reader's attention span. A reviewer should think not of his peers in the field but of the averagely intelligent but interested non-specialist (indeed, why should a peer really need to read a review?). The inspired teacher's gift for the helpful pause and reiteration of tricky concepts, aided by judicious use of tables and figures for relevant material, is likely to produce the best review.

A real requirement of a good review is that the author draws the strands of data together into a conclusion. The reader deserves a few "take home messages". At all costs, avoid the dreaded final sentence that simply states that all the present studies seem to be in conflict and that more research is needed. You will hear the collective groan of the readership when they get to the end only to find that they are, in reality, rather stuck in the middle. Remember that your review, like most of the really rewarding human endeavours, should end in some sort of climax.

13: The role of the editor

LEO VAN DE PUTTE, G SMITH

Introduction

The role of an editor in many respects is comparable with that of the conductor of an orchestra. The conductor is the person ultimately responsible for the objective – the best performance of the orchestra for the target audience. In that respect, the conductor is the main player, yet is totally dependent on and responsible for the optimal functioning of every link in the chain (the musicians), as well as for the total (the orchestra and its performance). In addition, responsibility for quality and its control implies (artistic) independence.

Very much the same applies to the editor of a scientific journal. He or she is responsible for fulfilment of the objectives of the journal, as well as for every step in the process involved in reaching that goal. The role of the editor can best be described as involving:

- meeting objectives of the journal
- overseeing the process and preconditions to reach these objectives
- avoiding common pitfalls.

The actual functioning of the editor can be influenced by a number of factors, including the organisation of the editorial team (centralised versus decentralised, see below), type of journal (for example, specialised versus general, weekly versus monthly), workload, and personal preference. Despite these differences, all editors have to face a number of core tasks, core processes, and responsibilities. For the sake of clarity, this chapter will describe the role of *a single* editor in chief as the ultimately responsible person, although we recognise that some journals have multiple editors, who function in a kind of dual management style.

The type of person that is editor of a (bio)medical journal is usually either a medical doctor – or at least someone who is familiar with the area of (bio)medicine of that particular journal. In addition, it is mandatory that the editor has some experience in publishing, preferably in the relevant medical field. It may also help if the editor is knowledgeable in the field and is seen by the profession as impartial. Although being an editor may be a full time job (especially for the weekly, general journals), for most specialist journals it is part time work.

Objectives of the journal

The final goal of every journal is to be a useful and almost inevitable means of communicating to the target readership. For this purpose, it is necessary to decide for what the journal stands. This may vary considerably. The typical journal dealt with in this chapter is a scientific, peer reviewed journal that frequently also includes material for (continued medical) education. When the journal is the official organ of a learned society, it may serve as a means of communication for that society. More generally oriented journals especially may include commentaries related to social and health policy issues. Unlike the other material, this need not necessarily be peer reviewed.

Responsibilities and qualities of the editor

It may seem superfluous to mention that the one person responsible for implementing the objectives is the editor. In fact, he or she is responsible for (at least):

- The whole content of the journal (including the advertisements!) – to ensure that it is of the highest possible standard.
- Steering and guiding the process needed to select the best manuscripts in an ethically sensible way and to present the content in the most appropriate manner. This also includes seeking the right balance in contributions (between clinical and non-clinical papers).

Ideally, an open selection procedure should be involved in appointing an editor, and the term of appointment should be fixed. I (Leo van de Putte) found it very helpful to have a detailed job description at the start of the job.

As there is no formal academic study to become an editor, and since many are part time editors, regular training is vital. As editor of the *Annals of the Rheumatic Diseases*, I (LvdP) appreciated (and found indispensable) the yearly editor's day and training courses offered to me to improve skills, discuss new developments (for instance, electronic publishing and its consequences and impact), and interact with other editors, the publisher, etc.

The journal's content

The content of a journal may vary according to the objectives of a journal (taking into account the kind of readership) and, in addition, is dependent on the nature of materials submitted. Of course the editor inevitably exercises considerable influence on the overall contents of the journal. Box 13.1 summarises sections that constitute the contents – the editor is responsible for an appropriate balance. Some journals may subclassify the sections according to individual diseases or techniques.

Box 13.1 Classification of contents of monthly scientific journals

- Editorial(s)
- Original articles

  - Clinical investigations
  - Laboratory investigations

- Short (rapid) communications
- Review article(s)
- Case report(s)
- Commentary
- Historical articles
- Apparatus
- Book reviews
- Correspondence
- Proceedings (or abstracts) of meetings of scientific societies

---

Editorials (leaders)

Editorials broadly fall into two categories:

- editorials on topical scientific, educational, or professional subjects
- editorials on the topic, or the specifics, of an accepted "in press" paper, to be published concurrently with that paper.

Original articles (extended reports)

Original articles are the mainstay of a scientific journal. These articles are the result of original work, usually in the field of clinical, translational, or basic (fundamental) research in (bio)medicine. In line with the objectives and scope of the journal, the editor may influence the topics, favouring particular areas in the field for instance, and influence the balance between clinical and non-clinical research.

Review articles

Review articles may be divided broadly into "educational" reviews, which inform the broad readership on the state of the art in a particular field or "scientific" reviews, which deal with a topic in depth and are meant for insiders of a particular field. Editors have great interest in review articles, because they are popular among the readership and may boost the impact factor.

Brief reports (concise reports, brief communications)

Brief reports include work that may be of interest but does not warrant publication as original work – either because of its incomplete nature (for example, an interesting pilot study) or simply because the work is too meagre for an extended report but nevertheless has some interesting aspects. This category is sometimes used for rapid publications.

Case reports

Case reports often present considerable difficulties for the editor. Criteria for acceptance vary among different journals, and the editor's opinion is quite important – ranging from refusing acceptance of any case report to being relatively liberal.

For acceptance in the *Annals of the Rheumatic Diseases*, case reports to be published as such (as a separate category, usually under the heading "concise reports") should be a unique problem, in terms of clinical presentation (diagnosis), treatment, or pathophysiology, and therefore may lead to further studies. Cases of lesser importance could be acceptable as a letter to the editor, and cases describing disease A plus an unrelated abnormality or disease B (usually being mere coincidence) are generally rejected.

Letters

This section consists of a mixture of short contributions and should be vivid. When outside the field of expertise of the editor, it should be peer reviewed. To avoid expansion of this section, it may be useful to have strict guidelines as to the length of the letters and the number of references, tables, and figures.

Correspondence

This is the forum for a lively and informative debate, and as such contributes considerably to the attractiveness and readability of the journal. Most of the correspondence relates to published articles in the journal. This section should be used for a real debate and not misused to bring similar cases or problems to the readers' attention. If so, it should be peer reviewed. Some journals now use the internet for rapid responses to published materials.

Book reviews and other categories

Book reviews are solicited by the editor. They are often popular among the readership. Other categories are numerous, such as "Viewpoint," "Special articles," "Vignettes," "Lesson of the month," etc.

Organisation

The editor as the central person in manuscript processing (and editing) has to deal with a large number of players in the game, which has become increasingly complex. Therefore, it is of vital importance that the role of the various players is well defined.

Most scientific journals have guidelines or instructions for authors and assessors (Box 13.2). As manuscripts are normally processed by a team (the editorial team) rather than by a single individual (the editor), it has become important to define the role of the others involved. As editor of the *Annals of the Rheumatic Diseases*, I (LvdP) found it very helpful to have job descriptions and/or defined responsibilities for the editorial assistant, associate editors, editorial board members, and, of course, the editor. Terms of office should be clearly indicated. A characteristic of a good journal is a regular influx and outflux of individuals who influence and shape the journal's content, especially the members of the editorial team.

Essentially two major methods are used to organise the editorial team: one being vertical and centralised, the other more horizontal and decentralised (Figure 13.1). In system A, the editor acts as the sole final conduit between acceptance of manuscripts in the editorial office and transmission to the technical editor of the publisher. In system B, several individuals may act as conduits between submission of manuscripts and transmission to the publisher. In this system, manuscripts that relate to particular subspecialties may be handled semi-independently by section editors – for example, in rheumatology, separate section editors may deal with manuscripts that cover the areas of inflammatory rheumatic diseases, soft tissue rheumatism, and pharmacotherapy, etc.

The two types of editorial organisation each have specific advantages and disadvantages. In the first system, greater uniformity of criteria exists for accepting and rejecting manuscripts and subediting. The disadvantage is a much higher workload for the single editor. In the second system, the workload is spread between several individuals, who may have greater expertise within their own specialised fields; however, the disadvantage is less uniformity of acceptance criteria and editing.

For specialised journals with a limited scope and number of submissions, system A may be preferable. Even for system B, it is preferable that there is at least one central mailbox, for the clarity of the authors, as well as for the editor to exercise their role as the central responsible person. Mixed systems do occur

Box 13.2 Guidelines for assessors*

1. The unpublished manuscript is a privileged document. Please protect it from any form of exploitation. Assessors are expected not to cite a manuscript or refer to the work it describes before it has been published and to refrain from using the information it contains for the advancement of their own research.

2. An assessor should consciously adopt a positive, impartial attitude towards the manuscript under review. Your position should be that of the author's ally, with the aim of promoting effective and accurate scientific communication.

3. If you believe that you cannot judge a given article impartially, please return the manuscript immediately to the editor with that explanation.

4. Reviews should be completed expeditiously, within 2–3 weeks. If you know that you cannot finish the review within the time specified, please inform the editor to determine what action should be taken.

5. An assessor should not discuss a paper with its author.

6. Please do not make any specific statement about the acceptability of a paper in your comments for transmission to the author, but advise the editor on the sheet provided.

7. In your review, please consider the following aspects of the manuscript as far as they are applicable:

   - importance of the question or subject studied
   - originality of the work
   - appropriateness of approach or experimental design
   - adequacy of experimental techniques (including statistics where appropriate)
   - soundness of conclusions and interpretation
   - relevance of discussion
   - clarity of writing and soundness of organisation of the paper.

8. In comments intended for the author's eyes, criticism should be presented dispassionately and abrasive remarks avoided.

9. Suggested revisions should be couched as such and not expressed as conditions of acceptance. On the sheet provided, please distinguish between revisions considered essential and those judged merely desirable.

10. Your criticisms, arguments, and suggestions about the paper will be most useful to the editor if they are documented carefully.

11. You are not asked to correct deficiencies of style or mistakes in grammar, but any help you can offer to the editor in this regard will be appreciated.

12. An assessor's recommendations are received gratefully by the editor, but as editorial decisions are based usually on evaluations derived from several sources, an assessor should not expect the editor to honour his or her every recommendation.

*These guidelines were prepared by the Council of Biology Editors.

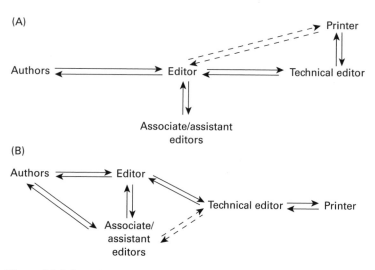

Figure 13.1 Organisation of the editorial team

and, in fact, may be desirable, depending on the objectives of the journal, its scope, and its workload.

Processing of manuscripts

Initial screening

Before seeking expert assessors' views on the manuscript, the editor should ensure that some basic formalities have been met.

- The manuscript should conform to the uniform requirements for manuscripts submitted to biomedical journals.[1] This agreement states that a manuscript must be accompanied by a covering letter signed by all authors of the manuscript. The letter should include information on prior or duplicate publication, or submission elsewhere, of any part of the work.
- A statement of financial or other relations that might lead to conflict of interests should be included.
- A statement that the manuscript has been read and approved by all authors should be included.

Box 13.3 Typical layout of a scientific manuscript

- Title page
- Summary, including keywords
- Introduction
- Methods
- Results
- Discussion
- Acknowledgements
- List of references
- Tables (including legends to tables)
- Legends to illustrations

- The name, address, telephone and fax numbers, and email address of the corresponding author should be noted.
- Each manuscript should be presented in the appropriate format. The typical layout for a scientific manuscript is shown in Box 13.3.

The editor also ensures initially that the content of the manuscript is appropriate for their particular journal. For example, if the journal is predominantly clinical, manuscripts that relate to basic laboratory investigations may be returned to the authors automatically without formal assessment.

Assessors' reports

After the initial screening, the editor seeks expert advice on the quality of the paper. Advice may be sought from one, two, three, or occasionally more expert assessors. The assessor is asked particularly if the work is original and if the methods are sufficiently accurate and reproducible to generate data on which sound conclusions may be based. Advice may be offered to the assessors in the form of standard guidelines (Box 13.2). Assessors may be asked to produce an anonymous report for transmission to the author and also to complete advisory guidelines confidential to the editor.

Review of assessors' reports

Armed with the assessors' advice and his or her own review of the manuscript, the editor may draw one of three conclusions.

- The manuscript is unacceptable for publication and is unlikely to be modified in such a way as to become acceptable for publication. Often the major reason for this decision is that the work is not original or that the methods of investigation are inappropriate or inaccurate. It may also become clear at this stage that the material is not appropriate for the particular journal.
- The manuscript is acceptable for publication either as it stands or with some minor modifications.
- The present manuscript is not acceptable for publication but it *might* become acceptable subject to modifications. In addition, guidance may be provided on the statistical handling of the data and editorial changes that may be required to produce conformity with the journal's style.

The revised manuscript

The editor may decide on his or her own initiative that the manuscript is acceptable for publication or, with the benefit of clarification of questions of originality or methods, that the paper clearly is quite unacceptable for publication. If additional expert advice is required, the editor may seek further reports from the original or additional assessors.

Editorial decision

It is important to emphasise that the assessors' reports represent only guidelines for the editor and they do not dictate the editor's course of action. Editorial decisions are based upon editorial policy, assessors' reports, the assessors' confidential comments to the editor, the editor's reading of the manuscript, the flow of manuscripts to the journal, and constraints imposed by the size of the journal. As only a relatively small proportion of manuscripts are immediately deemed acceptable or unacceptable for publication, the editor may rely heavily on his or her judgement of what represents an advance on our current state of knowledge and the degree to which confirmation is required. For example, when a new drug is introduced for the treatment of a particular disease, it is important that several centres, probably in different countries, provide confirmatory evidence of the pharmacological and therapeutic action of that drug. A time comes, however, when additional studies are not required and they may then be rejected.

Editing the manuscript

After an editor accepts a manuscript for publication, he or she may either edit the manuscript himself or herself or may pass it to an associate editor for this purpose. The process of editing follows certain principles.

- An attempt is made to shorten the manuscript without any loss of accuracy. Authors often repeat data in the results and discussion section of a manuscript. Repetition is common in a concluding paragraph or, indeed, if a summary is appended to the manuscript. A common form of repetition is where the same data appear in both tables and figures.
- Where manuscripts have emanated from non-English speaking countries, considerable effort may be required to correct English grammar.
- The editor may change phrases or sentences to standardise to a particular "house style."
- The references may be checked for accuracy and validity.
- The manuscript is standardised in respect of drug names, symbols, units, and abbreviations. Often, this work is undertaken by a professional subeditor (or technical editor).

Technical editing

After the editor finishes with the manuscript, it is passed with a disk to a technical editor, who edits the manuscript on screen and introduces notations needed to produce the correct fonts and lay out of the manuscript when it is produced by a computer controlled printing press.

Proof stage

Proofs from the printer are sent to the technical editor, the authors, and the editors – all of whom make corrections. These corrections are collated by the technical editor, who sends a corrected file to the printer.

Page proofs

Final page proofs are usually only seen by the editor and technical editor.

Publication

It will be clear from the foregoing that the process of publishing a scientific manuscript is complex and time consuming (Figure 13.2). For a monthly journal, therefore, it should be anticipated that many months will elapse between submission of a manuscript and its eventual publication.

Other published material

As the editor is responsible for assessing every word that appears in the journal, he or she needs to review all material, including advertisements, for both commercial and academic purposes. Commercial advertisements must be vetted closely to ensure that outrageous claims or inaccuracies are avoided and academic advertisements assessed for accuracy insofar as it is possible.

The editor's role: possible pitfalls

Editors play a central role in processing and editing a manuscript, and accepting or rejecting a paper is ultimately the editor's decision. For these reasons, he or she is also vulnerable. Authors and assessors may be dissatisfied with the editor's decisions or feel misinterpreted. Procedural, ethical, or privacy issues may have been overlooked, which may hurt not only the editor but also, of course, the journal. Editors will make mistakes. A few safeguards, however, may make the life of the editor more pleasant and safe, and his or her functioning more effective. Important in that respect are:

- The process of handling and editing should be transparent, and the individual responsibilities of the members of the editorial team should be well defined.
- As no one controls the editor, an open atmosphere should exist in the editorial team, allowing the editor to be easily

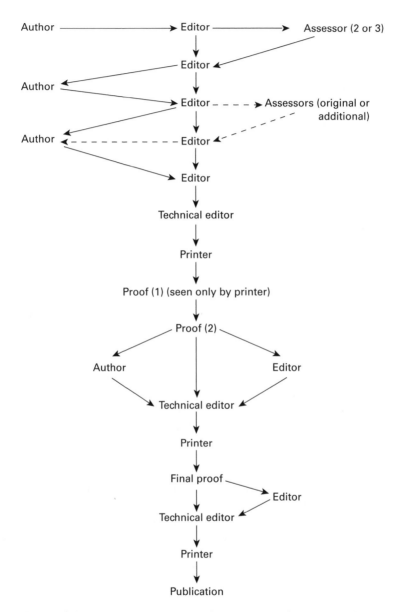

Figure 13.2 Stages in the progress of a manuscript from submission to publication

approached and open to constructive criticism. Regular meetings of, and discussions within, the editorial team may be valuable to and supportive for the editor.

- The editor should be keen on ethical and privacy issues. Many journals have signed up for the Committee on Publication Ethics (COPE). As many editors, especially those from specialist journals, are active in the research field, it is important to avoid even the slightest suspicion of conflict of interest. When the editor wishes to publish in his or her own journal, the manuscript should be dealt with by an acting editor, who ultimately and independently decides for or against publication.
- The editor should be independent, and this is an important issue for discussion before accepting the appointment. Influencing factors may be many and may come from various sources, including industry, the publisher, and learned societies. To discuss these items, meetings with other editors may be extremely useful.
- For the journal to maintain or improve its quality, two groups are of utmost importance: the authors who report their scientific work in manuscripts and the assessors who guarantee the quality of the peer review system. The editor should have good "bedside manners" when dealing with these important people. Reasonable complaints and remarks should be discussed and not dismissed. Assessors are probably the most essential and precious part of the whole manuscript processing procedure. Wise editors cherish the journal's assessors by not overloading them with papers, preferentially sending them papers within their field of expertise, and asking for a re-review of the revised manuscript by the assessor, if this was suggested. In our experience, assessors like to be asked whether they are willing to review a paper before it is sent to them.

Authors, of course, like a speedy process, and editors should be keen to monitor deadlines.

The future

Big changes in the recent past have occurred in manuscript processing and editing. Many journals are now doing the whole process electronically. Has this changed the life of the editor? In all probability it has. Some editors feel that the workload has increased; however, we are learning still. A definite advantage is that paper versions can be shortened, and therefore made more readable, when parts of the research that are of interest to a few (like extensive tables, databanks, appendices) can be put on the internet. Hopefully, electronic manuscript processing and editing will also speed up the time between manuscript submission and the final print version. Lively discussions have happened about the future of the paper versions of journals, but so far in the medical field, it seems that paper versions are still very popular. Another interesting point is the future of the peer review system. Although deemed an outdated system by some, most recognise that so far no better method exists for selection of manuscripts and quality control.

Reference

1 International Committee of Medical Journal Editors. Uniform requirements for manuscripts submitted to biomedical journals. *BMJ* 1988;**296**:401–5.

14: The role of the manuscript assessor

DOMHNALL MACAULEY

Introduction

You have been invited to review a paper. How can you help the editor, help the author, and get the most out of the experience? This chapter will look at the process of assessing papers: how your review can be of most value to the editor when he or she makes a decision about acceptance, rejection, or modification of a paper. If the decision is to reject, it will also help the author improve their paper for resubmission or future submission to another journal.

Every manuscript is important to the author. After endless hours of work – drafting and redrafting, negotiating with co-authors, checking tables and graphs, collating signatures, and massaging egos – the paper is finally completed and dispatched. And, so it arrives, with a polite note from the editor asking for your opinion.

Remember, you were once that author. If you have been asked to review a paper, you almost certainly will have had a successful research career and published a number of papers. You will remember how you sent off your first paper – nervous, anxious, and excited – and awaited the response and reviewer's opinion. You held the reviewer in such esteem, studying every word of their critique, analysing, and reanalysing their meaning. You grumbled if they did not understand your work, were thrilled at words of encouragement, were irritated if they did not seem up to date with the latest literature, and argued with their interpretation of the findings. So, be kind. It is a privilege to be asked to give an opinion on someone else's work, but with this invitation is a responsibility to do it well. By now, you may be a crusty old academic, well drilled in the ways of the world, and a little cynical. Many papers, however, are submitted by inexperienced authors setting out on their career. Although you will also be asked to review papers from experienced academics, you may be the assessor of a manuscript that is an author's first tentative step into the world of academia. Be helpful. Be the reviewer that you would have liked to review your first paper, and don't try to show how good you are. Be thorough and detailed. Above all, be fair and honest.

The role of reviewer gives little reward. Academic publishing is based on the generosity and altruism of researchers and requires a lot of work with little return. Most journals do not pay for reviews, and only recently has reviewing been recognised as a measure of academic esteem by universities. Good reviewing requires idealism and is a thankless task that takes time and effort to do well.[1] The primary reward is in the contribution the reviewer makes to the research community. It takes time, and reviewers, on average, spend 2·4 hours and review for 3·6 journals.[2]

Specialist versus generalist journals

Specialist and general journals may have different needs and expectations. In a specialist journal, the editor might ask two or more reviewers to assess a paper. The editor's knowledge is unlikely to span the entire breadth of the journal's range, so they need an expert opinion. The final decision on how to deal with the paper will be made by the editor alone, but having two or more opinions gives editors more confidence in their decision.

In large general journals, although an editor may not be expert in a particular field, there is likely to be a larger editorial faculty, with the paper passing through more than one editorial committee and seen by a number of assessors before subsequent acceptance or rejection. The reviewer's opinion carries considerable weight in the final decision in each case, but this opinion is only one part of the decision process and may be interpreted differently in different journals. Sometimes, although it is unusual, an editor may accept a paper of which the reviewer is unsupportive or reject a paper that the reviewer thinks should be published. In general, however, the reviewer does have considerable influence on the editorial decision.

The process

If the paper arrives by post, you should find a letter from the editor, a copy of the manuscript, and guidelines on what the editor would like in your review. You will be asked to give your opinion by a particular date, usually 3–4 weeks from receipt. It is often helpful to write a short note accepting the invitation to review, so the editorial assistant knows that the process is proceeding.

Electronic publishing has revolutionised paper handling, and an invitation to review often comes by email. You retrieve the abstract by a website or portal that allows you to decide if you know enough about the topic to undertake the review. The decision to review or not can be difficult. If you are not an expert in the field or are certain that you cannot complete the review in time, do let the editor know by return. If you have doubts about your time availability, respond immediately and decline – few people find that their days become less cluttered. If you can do it, however, please do. When you reply you will receive an electronic response, often instantaneous, thanking you and giving you access to the full paper. You may need Adobe Acrobat to read the paper; if you do not have this software, the journal will usually give you guidance on how to download it. After you have read the paper, you may have access to an electronic response form to submit your review. Alternatively, you may write your review on a word processor and attach or upload the file.

If you cannot complete the review in the time indicated, do let the editorial assistant and editor know as soon as possible. It is much better to know that a reviewer cannot help than for nobody to know what is happening. Yes, we have all been guilty – a paper for review sitting at the bottom of a pile of work, never quite making it to the top. Do try to complete it on time, otherwise the editorial assistant will have to chase you and it seems that the only way to get reviewers to produce on time is to remind them.[3]

Occasionally, you will be asked to review a paper where you know little about the topic. This may be a mistake on the part of the editor, who is misinformed about your field of expertise. Editors identify potential reviewers in many ways. Major journals have large electronic databases that can be searched with keywords identified from information that you, as a previous author or potential reviewer, have submitted yourself. Alternatively, the editor may have found your name on a database or identified you as an author on a paper on this or a related topic. Medline, for example, provides the email address of the corresponding author. This may not always be the best method to identify potential reviewers. Young ambitious academics tend to move jobs and universities fairly regularly, and the email address may be obsolete; interests change, so a paper published three years ago may reflect work carried out three or more years previously; or the corresponding author may not always be the overall expert behind the work. Mistakes happen, so be patient with editors, and do let us know as soon as possible if we have made an error!

On the other hand, an editor may have had difficulty identifying a reviewer with expertise in a particular specialist field and you may have been asked because you have a related interest. If, in these circumstances, you can write a review, please do. It might be a bit more difficult because you might have to read around the topic, but do give it some thought. Some papers appear jinxed, in that every potential reviewer approached declines and the editor is left with a list of refusals from reviewers and an increasingly anxious author who has waited a long time for an opinion.

And, please forgive the poor editor who mistakenly invites you to review a paper you have submitted yourself. Yes, by searching topic codes, I identified the perfect reviewer, someone who had written extensively on the subject. I should have checked the author list!

The best and the worst reviews

The perfect review does not exist. Neither of course, does the perfect paper. But, the best review is one that informs both the editor and the author of the limitations and possible improvements to a paper.

The editor, primarily, needs to know if a paper is suitable for publication and how it can be improved. If the work has fatal flaws, usually in relation to the methods, this makes the decision to reject much easier. If the paper could be acceptable with modification, the editor needs to know if this can be done. Minor problems can be corrected easily.

The best reviewer reads around the topic. With such easy access to electronic databases at hospitals, at universities, and on home computers, an editor expects the assessor to do a brief search of the literature to be able to comment on the originality of the work.

No strict guidelines exist on the structure of a review, but a general consensus seems to have evolved that divides the review into three parts. The first part is usually a general comment on the paper – its originality, importance, and validity. The second part deals with major problems, and the third section lists minor problems. This structure can be used in any review and is a delight to the editor and author.

A helpful review begins with a short summary that places the paper in context and essentially answers the twin questions: is it new and is it true?

The reviewer should indicate if, in the context of their specialist knowledge, the subject matter or research question is of sufficient importance and novelty that it merits publication. The assessor should also know enough about the journal to know whether the style and content fits within the remit or range of interest of the journal.

Example

Summary

This is an interesting and well written paper on peer review. The authors have identified an important research question and have addressed it in an organised and well structured paper. The paper is well written and fits with the style of the *Journal of Medical Writing*. I have some major concerns about the sampling method and some minor concerns about the accuracy of writing.

The second section of the review might highlight major criticisms of the paper. It will address the relevance and appropriateness of the introduction, problems identified in the methods, the accuracy of the results, the interpretation of these results in the discussion, and the objectivity and validity of the conclusion. Each identified problem should be referenced immediately to the text of the paper by the page number, paragraph number, and line number. Direct quotations included in the review should be in parentheses. This allows both the editor and the author to look to the text and locate the problem immediately. Major criticisms should be recognisable as fatal flaws that would prevent publication of the paper.

Example

Major criticisms

Page 2, paragraph 2, line 3. The authors describe their sampling method. Allocation by day of arrival of a manuscript is not an acceptable method of randomisation in a randomised controlled trial.
Page 2, paragraph 2, line 7. The authors do not identify the inclusion and exclusion criteria.

The third section lists minor criticisms, and it may include advice on possible improvements to the introduction, suggestions for additional references, and comments on the context of the paper and errors in spelling and grammar.

Example

Minor criticisms

Page 1, paragraph 3, line 2. The introduction covers the literature appropriately, although the authors may like to look at two other papers on randomised controlled trials (Godlee *et al.* and van Royen *et al.*).
Page 1, paragraph 3, line 4. Misspelling of the word trial – spelt "trail."

Case reports are treated differently. Some journals publish case reports regularly and others only in special circumstances. The *BMJ*, for example, does not publish case reports unless they are submitted as a "lesson of the week." The key issue with a case report is its originality. The author genuinely believes that theirs is an original observation, so reviewers should check the literature. Similar cases may have been reported in a different field, language, or country and have not been reported previously in this specialty or geographical location. Different editors use different criteria, and the role of the reviewer is to provide enough information to allow the editor to make a decision.

Improving the quality

The peer review process has evolved as a method of objective selection on scientific merit. It is, however, at best, an inexact science, and little indicates that peer review gives a better decision in the end. Indeed, a recent systematic review from the international Cochrane Collaboration (http://www.nelh.nhs.uk) concluded that little hard evidence showed that peer review improved the quality of published biomedical research.[4] It is also difficult to measure the quality of peer review, with little agreement on measures of quality.[5]

One alternative to aim for is blinded review, but complete blinding is difficult and 23–42% of reviewers not told the identity of authors were able to identify them. Papers nearly always include some reference to the location or special nature of the population being examined. Most researchers know the other researchers in a specialist field and can often identify their work.

In the interests of honesty and transparency, many journals now opt for open peer review. In this system, both the author and the reviewer know each other's identity. Some argue that this may make reviewers less likely to give an incisive and critical review, but it also protects the author from the unscrupulous reviewer.

A number of randomised controlled trials have been conducted on blinding or open peer review.[6,7] In a recent article in *JAMA*,[8] Fiona Godlee, one of the key researchers in the field, puts the case that open review is superior ethically to anonymous reviews and that open review increases the accountability of the reviewers, with less scope for biased or unjustified judgements or misappropriation of data under the cloak of anonymity.

Open review does have possible disadvantages. It may increase the number of reviewers who decline to review, the likelihood that reviewers will recommend acceptance, and the time taken to produce a report. It is also possible that junior reviewers would be less likely to give an honest criticism of work by senior colleagues. Threats – overt or covert – and bullying by more senior academics are possible. In order to protect reviewers, when the *BMJ* introduced its open peer review,[9] it also introduced a system of anonymous notification of intimidation of reviewers. They termed this the yellow card system, because of its similarity to the drug adverse reaction notification system in the United Kingdom.

With open review, the author may take their complaint directly to the reviewer, rather than going through the editorial process. This, of course, is inappropriate. In such cases, the reviewer should not respond directly but should contact the editor. This allows both parties to take a step back from direct conflict and the editor to settle any differences.

Bias – conscious or subconscious – is always a possibility. A reviewer may be tempted to favour a former collaborator's work or may have a tendency to be more critical of the work of a competitor. Indeed, the reviewer may, because of their specialist knowledge, know more about the potential pitfalls and mistakes involved in research in a particular area.

If you would like to find out more about improving the quality of your peer review, you may like to look at guidance on the website of the World Association of Medical Editors (http://www.wame.org/syllabus.htm#reviewers and http://www.wame.org/wamestmt.htm).

Dealing with an appeal

The tendency is increasing for authors to appeal an editor's decision. This creates a dilemma. Everyone makes mistakes, and editors, perhaps more than most, are aware of the weaknesses of the peer review process and acutely aware that the system can fail. If an editor has any doubt that a paper may have been rejected unfairly, they will usually re-examine the decision. That process often includes asking for a further review. In such cases, the editor will usually send all the correspondence, together with the previous review(s), to the new assessor and will ask for a further opinion. The assessor should go through exactly the same process of assessing the paper on its merits. The final decision will be with the editor, but as the reviewer, you are the consultant advisor, whose advice helps that decision.

Referee, reviewer, or assessor

The deliberate use of the term assessor or reviewer in this chapter is an attempt to move away from the term referee. Sometimes assessors find the task difficult and are uncomfortable making decisions about the work of their peers. It helps to remember, however, that the final decision is with the editor, and it is their responsibility. The use of the term referee can be misleading, because it is the editor who must make the decision. Your role, as reviewer, is to give an honest assessment of the value of a piece of work in the context of your knowledge, experience, and your brief review of the relevant literature.

Improving the quality of the review

Research suggests that the best peer reviewers are aged under 40 years, trained in epidemiology or statistics, and live in North America. Little evidence shows that the quality of reviews can be improved,[10] and, any effect of training is negative. The quality of a review depends greatly on how much time and effort the reviewer is prepared to invest.

Do authors care? It is difficult to know, but one study of 897 corresponding authors of the *Annals of Emergency Medicine*, with a 64% response rate, showed modest satisfaction with peer review.[11] Those authors whose papers were accepted were most satisfied with peer review, and authors of rejected manuscripts were dissatisfied both with the time taken to decision and the communication from the editor. Authors were happy if their paper was accepted irrespective of review quality.

Conflict of interest

Reviewers do have an ethical responsibility. Assessors are chosen because of their interest in the particular field, so you may find yourself appraising the work of your former colleagues or your competitors. If this creates a conflict of interest, do let the editor know. The peer review process is based entirely on trust. It depends on your integrity and, just as you would expect an honest and true assessment of your work, so do your colleagues – even if they are your competitors. Authors sometimes submit their manuscripts with a request that the editor does not use certain reviewers, who they feel may not give a fair assessment. Although we expect assessors to have the utmost integrity, most editors would consider such as request to be reasonable.

You also have a responsibility to maintain the integrity of the peer review system, however, and, if you think an author could possibly have any concern about your independence, do contact the editor. On the other hand, sometimes you may be the only person qualified to review a paper. Disclosure is the best protection against an accusation of conflict of interest. If you inform the editor and try to give an honest appraisal of the paper, you have done everything that you can do. The editor can then disclose to the author, if necessary, that you highlighted a potential conflict of interest.

You also have a responsibility for intellectual integrity; you must not use other people's ideas. It does happen – and can happen even subconsciously – so it is important to be on your guard.

A fascinating example of conflict of interest is described on the website of the World Association of Medical Editors (http://www.wame.org/conflict.htm). It was submitted anonymously by an editor and discussed at the Fourth International Congress on Peer Review in Barcelona in September 2001. The case was presented to the audience by Michael Callaham of the WAME Ethics Committee and was discussed by an expert panel, consisting of Richard Smith (*BMJ*), Richard Horton (*Lancet*), and Frank Davidoff (*Annals of Internal Medicine*).

Research misconduct

You may, at times, as an assessor, have doubts about a paper. It may be that you doubt the figures, the tables, the complete reporting of results, manipulation of sampling, etc. If you suspect research misconduct, it is important that you bring your doubts to the attention of the editor. You could be wrong, however, so this must be done in a subtle and sensitive manner.

The editor has a number of options in such cases, but the most likely is that he or she will ask the author to supply the original data, information on sampling arrangements, a copy of the ethical approval, etc. This may uncover a mistake, a misreport, an error of judgement, or a deliberate attempt to mislead. As a reviewer, it is important not to make a judgement or accusation without serious consideration and a degree of certainty. If there is a problem or doubt, the editor may ask the Committee on Publication Ethics (COPE) to consider the case.[12]

If you are concerned about duplicate or "salami" publication, it is helpful if you send copies of other relevant papers so the editor can identify the degree of overlap. Academic departments are under huge amounts of pressure to publish as many papers as possible, and there may be the temptation to try to split a piece of work into multiple manuscripts to maximise the number of publications and increase the maximum number of papers on curriculum vitae. In the current academic climate, such salami publishing is understandable but inappropriate. It clutters up the literature and makes it difficult to identify the true message in any piece of work.

Conclusion

It is an honour and a privilege to be asked to give a prepublication opinion on a colleague's work. The academic world depends on the altruism of researchers to ensure the continued existence of peer review. There is also a responsibility to do it well, however. Try to invest the time and effort into providing the type of review you would like from an assessor asked to review your work.

References

1 Goldbeck-Wood S. What makes a good reviewer of manuscripts. *BMJ* 1998;**316**:86.
2 Yankaur A. Who are the peer reviewers and how much do they review. *JAMA* 1990;**263**:1338–40.
3 Pitkin RM, Burmeister LF. Prodding tardy reviewers. *JAMA* 2002;**287**: 2794–5.
4 White C. Little evidence for effectiveness of scientific peer review. *BMJ* 2003;**326**:241.
5 Jefferson T, Wager E, Davidoff F. Measuring the quality of editorial peer review. *JAMA* 2002;**287**:2786–90.
6 Godlee F, Cale CR, Martyn CN. Effect on the quality of peer review of blinding reviewers and asking them to sign their reports: a randomised controlled trial. *JAMA* 1998;**280**:237–40.

7 Van Royen S, Godlee F, Evans S, Smith R, Black N. Effect of blinding and unmasking on the quality of peer review: a randomised controlled trial. *JAMA* 1998;**280**:234–7.
8 Godlee F. Making reviewers visible. Openness, accountability, and credit. *JAMA* 2002;**287**:2762–5.
9 Smith R. Opening up *BMJ* peer review. *BMJ* 1999;**318**:4–5.
10 Callaham M, Knopp RK, Gallagher EJ. Effect of written feedback by editors on quality of reviews. *JAMA* 2002;**287**:2781–3.
11 Weber EJ, Katz PP, Waeckerle JF, Callaham MI. Author perception of peer review. *JAMA* 2002;**287**:2790–3.
12 Smith R. Misconduct in research: editors respond. *BMJ* 1997;**315**:201–2.

15: What a publisher does

ALEX WILLIAMSON

Congratulations! Your paper has been accepted for publication.

At this point, the author may have his or her first contact with the publisher. This should be a rewarding and pleasant experience, but many authors have only a vague notion of what a publisher actually does.

Authors write and the publishers provide the means for those authors to reach their audiences – traditionally via a print medium. Now we also have the means to reach a potentially much larger and more international audience via the internet. The services that a journal publishing house offers fall into a number of broad categories: editorial, production, sales and marketing, subscription fulfilment, distribution, and finance. An author will have no direct contact with some of the latter categories, but they nevertheless are essential to the business. Each category is dependent on the others, and all work closely together.

Editorial

Typically two main functions exist within the editorial department – managing and commissioning, and copyediting.

Managing and commissioning editors

Managing and commissioning editors (also called publishing managers, acquisitions editors, or sponsoring editors) are the publishers' representatives to journal editors, learned societies, and authors. The main function of a managing editor is the care of the existing list of journals. This consists of financial management, liaison with the learned society (if one is involved), overseeing the duties of the copy editor, editorial assistants, both online and print production, advertisement sales, marketing, subscription fulfilment and distribution, and – last but by no means least – liaison with and support of the journal editors. These editors are a rare breed of dedicated professionals who are often full time clinicians, academics, or both. For modest or no reward, they devote many hours to editorial work and need strong support from the publisher.

Managing editors will also receive new journal proposals, seek specialist opinion via both questionnaires and personal contacts, analyse and research the market, cost the proposal, and, finally, present it to their management. The rejection rate for new journal proposals is very high indeed – roughly speaking, only one in 10 proposals will be successful. A new journal launch requires a large investment from the publisher, so a decision to launch is never taken lightly.

The managing editor will meet the editor regularly, offer advice on publishing practice, and help to train support staff for the editorial office. In recent times, the managing editor has had to learn a new skill: they need to be up to date with internet developments.

Almost all journals now have an online presence as well as a print version. The online version may be a simple listing of tables of contents and abstracts. Increasingly, however, journals' websites are much more sophisticated, with html and pdf text, search engines, substantial back archives, subject collections, data supplements, hyperlinks to other useful sites, and much, much more. The managing editor should be able to recommend new functionalities, suggest the uploading of additional data to enhance the site, and make it a much more useful and comprehensive resource than the print version.

The whole peer review process is also in the process of change. For some years now, most journals have used a software package to administer the peer review procedure for commissioned articles and submitted unsolicited manuscripts. The editorial office was often based at the editor's main place of work or at the publishing house. Most journals would employ a full or part time editorial assistant(s), whose role was to administer that process, chase recalcitrant reviewers, and deal with all the editor's correspondence with authors, editorial board members, and reviewers. Generally speaking, these editorial assistants would be recruited, funded, and trained by the publisher. The internet is revolutionising the peer review process, and the signs are that it is speeding it up too. More and more journals are migrating to a web based manuscript submission and peer review system. This means that the journal is "open for business" 24 hours a day, seven days a week, and it is accessible from anywhere in the world that has internet access. It is now almost irrelevant as to where the editorial office is situated. Although postage and stationery costs will fall, telephone costs may soar – particularly for those using a dial up modem.

Once a manuscript is accepted for publication, the editor or editorial assistant will send it as an electronic file to the publisher, where it will receive the attention of the copy editor.

Copy editors

Copy editors (also called technical editors, subeditors, or production editors) provide the main link between an author and the publisher. The copy editor will prepare the accepted manuscript for publication in print and on the web. Most copy editing is now done on screen with the author's own word processed file. These electronic files will then be translated automatically into the appropriate format for the print and electronic versions of the journal. Copy editors have learned new skills and, in many cases, will be adding tagging and codes to the word processed author file so that the page make up programme can operate seamlessly and take in the artwork, figures, and tables, which will also have been generated electronically. The copy editor will also scrutinise the tables and illustrations.

Copy editors adapt the manuscript to the "house style" of the journal. They are concerned with details of style and ensure that spelling, grammar, punctuation, capitalisation, and mathematical conventions follow approved practice. They also look for accuracy and consistency. They pick up loose ends, discrepancies, omissions, and contradictions. Substantive queries may be referred back to the author and editor at this stage. More often, the problems identified are minor and will appear as queries to the author on the proof. Copy editors will suggest relettering and redrawing of illustrations where necessary and will size them and place them appropriately in the text.

Copy editors liaise with the supplier and ensure that proofs are distributed quickly to authors and editors. They will read the proofs and collate any corrections received from authors and editors. Only in exceptional circumstances are authors allowed to make major changes to their papers at this stage, and the copy editor will refer substantive author corrections for the editor's approval.

Copy editors work to tight schedules and often need to remind authors to return proofs promptly. Again, technology is helping to speed up the process. Many publishers require their suppliers to provide proofs in a pdf format, so that they can be emailed to authors as an attachment.

In collaboration with the editor and the advertisement department, copy editors make up the contents of each issue and pass final proofs for press. At this stage, the publishing process passes to the production department.

Copyright

Either at acceptance of the manuscript for publication or at the proof stage, the author may be required to assign copyright to the journal. Publishers are much better able to defend copyright than individual authors and will act on their behalf. However, practices are changing. Now, many journals simply require that authors grant them an exclusive licence to publish their article in print and on the web. Authors retain copyright and are able to use their own material freely elsewhere.

Competing interests

Some journals have been sensitised to the potential for competing interests to compromise the validity of a study and may require the author to complete a declaration. Competing interests may exist when professional judgement about a primary interest (such as patients' welfare or the validity of research) may be influenced by a secondary interest (such as financial gain or personal rivalry). It may arise for the authors of a journal article when they have a financial interest that may influence – probably without their knowing – their interpretation of their results or those of others. Many publishers may require authors to complete a competing interest declaration.

Offprints and reprints

Offprints are extra copies of the articles that are printed at the same time as the journal issue. Some publishers offer a quantity of these gratis to the author. This used to be a very popular service for authors, but the ease of photocopying has almost eliminated the need. Many publishers have now substituted provision of a free copy of the relevant journal issue to the corresponding author instead of providing free offprints. Other publishers will offer the author the opportunity to purchase a quantity of reprints at cost. In addition, some journals provide a pdf of the article to the author or free access to that article on the journal's website.

Production

Very few journals now use conventional typesetters, but they instead send their edited electronic files to an originating house (usually but not always part of a major printing house). Here the edited text files are married with the tables, figures, and illustrations, and the article is proofed. After final approval for publication and the journal issue has been made up, the online and print versions take different routes.

The print production staff will choose appropriate printers for the journal, bearing in mind the budget, print run, schedule, and use of colour illustrations and advertisements. They choose and purchase text paper and cover boards. The production department is responsible for schedules, obtains estimates, and controls costs. It keeps abreast of the latest advances in print and bind technology, and it will advise editorial colleagues on appropriate new means of production that will benefit the journal in terms of schedule, cost, and appearance. Overall, the production team is responsible for the look of the journal, its cost effective production on schedule, and its delivery for onward distribution to subscribers.

Most publishers have chosen a third party for hosting and maintaining their journal websites. On completion of an issue, the electronic files are sent to the hosting service for the addition of further programming before uploading. Many journal websites also have sections that are under the control of the editor and publisher to facilitate the addition of extra material and hyperlinks.

Fulfilment and distribution

The average peer reviewed journal's circulation is subscription based, usually on an annual basis. Again, the availability of online versions of most journals has given more options but undoubtedly has made the entire process more complex. Some publishers "bundle" their subscriptions so customers pay a single price and receive both a print version and access to the online version. Others have "unbundled" and offer a choice between print or online versions. All manner of pricing models exist.

By and large, subscribers fall into four main categories.

1 Institutional or library subscriptions at the full price subscription rate. Most of these sales are handled via subscription agents, who make the librarians' jobs much simpler. Librarians will probably deal with only one agent for the thousands of subscriptions they purchase. The agent will consolidate these orders and deal with the individual publishers, quite often using computers to facilitate the transfer of orders. For this service, the publishers give agents a discount.
2 Personal subscriptions at a discounted subscription rate.
3 Member subscriptions. Often a journal will be owned by or published in association with a learned society. The annual membership subscription may include an automatic subscription to the society's journal.
4 Free and exchange subscriptions. The editor and editorial board will normally receive free copies. Copyright legislation decrees that journal issues must be deposited in the British Library and several other major libraries. Subscriptions are given to the large abstracting and indexing services such as *Index Medicus, Current Contents*, and *Excerpta Medica*.

All of these groups expect to receive the journal regularly and on time, and subscribers need to be reminded each year to renew their subscriptions. Most subscription fulfilment systems are computer based and will generate mailing labels sorted into postal categories to a defined schedule. In many cases, these mailing labels will be despatched directly to the printer, who will arrange onward posting to subscribers. In other cases, publishers will handle all distribution from their own warehouses. Overseas consignments are often sent in bulk by air to a mailing house, which then organises onward distribution by that country's mail service. The warehouse will store additional copies of the journal to fulfil claims for missing issues, back orders, and single copy sales.

Sales and marketing

The main source of revenue for a journal comes from the sale of paid subscriptions. There are other sources, however, and I will deal with these before returning to the subscription area.

Advertising sales

The higher circulation general and specialist clinical journals enjoy substantial revenues from the sale of display advertising space in each issue. The major space buyers are the pharmaceutical companies, but equipment manufacturers and publishers also use journals to advertise their products.

The advertisement sales team not only maintains close links with agencies and companies, but it also liaises with the editorial team. A strong editorial policy on the percentage of advertisement versus editorial pages is needed, together with a strict code on the permitted content of advertisements and their location in comparison with editorial pages. Many journals operate a strict policy of not allowing advertisement sales in relation to editorial copy, and often editors will be allowed the right of veto. Despite these safeguards, editors and publishers are often criticised about the content and placement of advertisements. Nevertheless, advertisements can provide a useful service to the reader and certainly support the journal financially. The sale of advertising space to online versions is still in its infancy, and there is uncertainty as to whether or not it is sustainable in the long term.

Reprint sales

Reprint sales can be a considerable source of revenue, particularly where papers are reporting the results of clinical trials or new indications for an existing drug. Reprints should not be confused with offprints. Offprints are printed simultaneously with the journal and are primarily given free or sold at cost to authors. Reprints are produced later, usually in bulk, are of necessity more expensive, and appeal to the commercial sector.

Rights

The marketing of a journal involves not only the sale of subscriptions but also the sale of subsidiary rights. These may take the form of translation rights, rights to produce an English language edition in a slightly modified form for a foreign market, or rights to produce cheap reprints in countries where purchasing power is low. Additionally, journals will sell the rights to host their content or header information to third party aggregators such as Ovid or Ingenta.

Bulk and single copy sales and online sales

Occasionally, a journal will publish a special issue or supplement on a particular "hot" topic, and this may attract bulk sales from a commercial organisation or single copy sales to individuals. Many journal websites also carry "pay per view" or "pay for access." This functionality facilitated by e-commerce packages allows non-subscribers to access particular articles or to have access to the whole site for a period for payment of a modest sum.

Subscription sales and marketing

When a new journal is launched, the circulation climbs steadily and then plateaus as the journal becomes established in its specialty. Some people are of the opinion that once a journal has reached its plateau, it is no longer necessary to continue active promotion. Not so! Every year, an established journal will lose some 10% of its circulation because of consolidation of library collections, budgetary restrictions, or simply a change in the direction of research in the institution.

To maintain its circulation, a journal needs to be promoted to pick up new subscribers to replace those that have been lost.

In collaboration with the subscription and fulfilment department, the lapsed subscribers will be encouraged actively to renew their subscriptions, and ultimately they will receive a questionnaire that can provide valuable information to editorial colleagues.

The marketing department is concerned with promotion material, publicity, and advertising. It devises campaigns to promote each journal, and it designs, writes, and produces leaflets and catalogues that are sent by direct mail to specialists and librarians worldwide. Apart from direct mail, journals are promoted via advertisements in other relevant high circulation journals and displays at appropriate specialty meetings and symposia.

As in every other facet of publishing, the internet also has changed the role of the marketing executive. Although most of the activities outlined above continue, often in a lesser form, the marketeers now have a much more direct role in selling site licences for online products direct to librarians or to consortia (groups of libraries that come together to increase their buying power). Some publishers now host library advisory groups where publisher and librarian can exchange views and take heed of each others' needs.

The internet is now used as a very effective marketing tool that can reach a large target audience very cheaply, and, if managed well, it can provide useful details of the customers who visit the site. Most of the major publishers have websites that act as a showcase for their publications. Many of these sites will also enable e-commerce so that orders can be placed and paid for directly. Targeted email campaigns seem more effective than relying on the old stalwart of direct mail shots.

Finance

The members of staff of the finance department have a number of roles – all of them concerned with money! They raise invoices, control cash flow, maintain records, and pay suppliers. The management accountant will provide monthly accounts to the senior management and will play an integral part in the constitution of annual budgets and longer term strategic planning.

Conclusion

The role of the publisher has been compared with a variety of functions, few of them favourable. We have been told we are parasites or denigrated as middlemen who come between the author and the reader. Perhaps we are best regarded as catalysts. We facilitate the communication between the authors and their readers. Even with the arrival of the internet, we are still needed to provide an efficient means to sift through, sort, and disseminate the fruits of your labours.

16: Who should be an author?

RICHARD HORTON

Regrettably this question is impossible to answer. Five years ago, I could have confidently referred you to the standard definition provided by the International Committee of Medical Journal Editors (otherwise known as the Vancouver Group) (Box 16.1).[1] All was clear back then. The criteria that had to be satisfied for you to qualify as an author (to be, shall we say, Vancouver Group positive) were unambiguous.

And they needed to be. Authorship is the currency of academic life. Citation provides the intellectual credit that fuels promotion and career success; it gives an independent estimate of a researcher's contribution to science. Authorship is the foundation of our system for judging academic value and assigning reward.

Before I ruin this picture of serene harmony, I should point out that most biomedical journals adhere to the Vancouver Group definition.[2] Their editors will require you to be Vancouver Group positive. In other words, to confirm in either a covering letter or a separate signed statement that you fulfil the Vancouver definition. You are likely to say you do even if you know that you or a co-author do not. To provide your signature confirming that you qualify as an author is something you do automatically, perhaps without even thinking very much about the implications of what you are doing.

Nowadays, though, the certainty that editors of leading medical journals once possessed lies in shreds. Our happy consensus has been destroyed. Following a conference on authorship in biomedical science, held in Nottingham, UK, in 1996,[3] first *The Lancet*[4] and then the *BMJ*[5] abandoned the Vancouver Group definition (although their editors are part of the Group). In its place we put the concept of contributorship,

---

Box 16.1 How to be a Vancouver Group positive author

All persons designated as authors should qualify for authorship. Each author should have participated sufficiently in the work to take public responsibility for the content.

Authorship credit should be based only on substantial contributions to: (1) conception and design or analysis and interpretation of data; (2) drafting the article or revising it critically for important intellectual content; and (3) final approval of the version to be published. Conditions 1, 2, and 3 must all be met. Participation solely in the acquisition of funding or the collection of data does not justify authorship. General supervision of the research group is not sufficient for authorship. Any part of an article critical to its main conclusions must be the responsibility of at least one author.

Editors may ask authors to describe what each contributed; this information may be published.

Increasingly, multicentre trials are attributed to a corporate author. All members of the group who are named as authors, either in the authorship position below the title or in a footnote, should fully meet the above criteria for authorship. Group members who do not meet these criteria should be listed, with their permission, in the acknowledgements or in an appendix.

The order of authorship should be a joint decision of the co-authors. Because the order is assigned in different ways, its meaning cannot be inferred accurately unless it is stated by the authors. Authors may wish to explain the order of authorship in a footnote. In deciding on the order, authors should be aware that many journals limit the number of authors listed in the table of contents and that the US National Library of Medicine (NLM) lists in Medline only the first 24 plus the last author when there are more than 25 authors.

---

an idea first described by Fotion and Conrad[6] but developed more fully by Drummond Rennie and colleagues.[7,8] This shift away from traditional notions of authorship is the most important recent crack to appear in the architecture of academia. It has the potential to threaten the entire structure of modern science. Why? And where does that leave you, someone who simply wants to get your work published?

First, most scientists ignore editors and most so called authors are likely to test Vancouver Group negative. For example, Shapiro et al.[9] found that a quarter of the "authors" they surveyed contributed nothing or to only one aspect of the published work.

Eastwood *et al.*[10] discovered that a third of the US postdoctoral fellows they questioned were happy to list someone as an author even if he or she did not deserve it, provided that the inclusion of their name would make publication more likely. Given this widespread cynicism about the meaning of authorship, to cling to a definition that no one uses seems crazy.

There is a second, more sensitive reason for questioning our existing beliefs about authorship. Several recent instances of scientific fraud[11,12] have revealed that the flipside of authorship *credit* – namely, authorship *responsibility* – is often overlooked. When individual researchers have their names listed on the byline of a paper, it can be difficult to dissect out who did what if an aspect of the work is questioned. Instances of fabrication or falsification of data have revealed the importance of assigning the precise and explicit parts played by individual investigators in a research project.

These two forces make it hard to resist two ensuing interpretations. First, that researchers should be allowed to list whoever they wish on the byline of a paper, Vancouver Group positive or negative. And second, that editors should ask for and publish a clear description of the contributions made by the authors. Rigid, unenforceable, and widely ignored definitions should be abandoned. This is the new policy of the *BMJ*[5] and *The Lancet*[4] The *BMJ* has gone further than *The Lancet* and asks each group of contributors to select one or more guarantors who will take overall responsibility for the integrity of the entire work.

The reaction to contributorship has been mixed. At *The Lancet*, we have found that most authors readily accept the idea that contributors should be cited at the end of each paper (Box 16.2). But some have voiced concerns that unethical authorship practices – inappropriate credit in the form of guest authors or the unacknowledged contributions of ghost authors – are likely to continue.[13]

Still, other journals are likely to follow the move to contributorship. Even if contributor lists are not always embraced, the principle of complete disclosure and personal responsibility is accepted.[14] You need to be aware which journals prefer traditional Vancouver Group positive authors and which prefer contributors. For all practical purposes, you can freely ignore the rules set by the former group. Everybody else does.

An additional issue that also defies easy rules is the acknowledgement section of your paper. Whom you choose to

---

Box 16.2 An example of contributorship

Byline: A, B, C, D, E, F, G, H

Contributors: A carried out the trial, helped in data analysis, and wrote the paper. B was involved in design, implementation, and data analysis, and contributed to the writing of the paper. C was involved in execution of the trial, data management and analysis, and quality assurance of the turnip assay. D was involved in trial execution and data entry, management analysis, and quality assurance. E was involved in trial execution and data management with emphasis on analysis. F and G were involved in the design and contributed to the writing of the paper. H was involved in the design, implementation, analysis, and biochemical interpretation, and contributed to the writing of the paper.

[Guarantors: A and H]

Box 16.3 Acknowledgements according to Vancouver

At an appropriate place in the article (the title page footnote or an appendix to the text; see the journal's requirements), one or more statements should specify: (1) contributions that need acknowledging but do not justify authorship, such as general support by a departmental chair; (2) acknowledgements of technical help; (3) acknowledgements of financial and material support, which should specify the nature of the support; and (4) relationships that may pose a conflict of interest.

Persons who have contributed intellectually to the paper but whose contributions do not justify authorship may be named and their function or contribution described – for example, "scientific adviser", "critical review of study proposal", "data collection", or "participation in clinical trial". Such persons must have given their permission to be named. Authors are responsible for obtaining written permission from persons acknowledged by name, because readers may infer their endorsement of the data and conclusions.

Technical help should be acknowledged in a paragraph separate from that acknowledging other contributions.

---

thank can be impossible to separate from whom you choose to cite as an author on the byline. Not surprisingly, the Vancouver Group has something to say about acknowledgements (Box 16.3). The likelihood is that contributor lists and acknowledgements will eventually fuse and the whole subject of academic reward based on research contributions will be overhauled.[15]

Given this confusing state, there is only one rule to bear in mind when deciding who is an author, a contributor, a guarantor, or an acknowledgee. Decide who is to be what *before* you start your study. Most authorship disputes arise when the work is completed and a paper has to be written. Then comes the jostling for a place (and position) on the byline. Primary prevention is always better in the end.

References

1 International Committee of Medical Journal Editors. Uniform requirements for manuscripts submitted to biomedical journals. *Ann Intern Med* 1997;**126**:36–47.
2 Parmley WW. Authorship: taking the high road. *J Am Coll Cardiol* 1997;**29**:702.
3 Horton R, Smith R. Signing up for authorship. *Lancet* 1996;**347**:780.
4 Horton R. The signature of responsibility. *Lancet* 1997;**350**:5–6.
5 Smith R. Authorship is dying: long live contributorship. *BMJ* 1997;**315**:686.
6 Fotion N, Conrad CC. Authorship and other credits. *Ann Intern Med* 1984;**100**:592–4.
7 Rennie D, Flanagin A. Authorship! Authorship! Guests, ghosts, grafters, and the two-sided coin. *JAMA* 1994;**278**:469–71.
8 Rennie D, Yank V, Emanuel L. When authorship fails: a proposal to make contributors accountable. *JAMA* 1997;**278**:579–85.
9 Shapiro SW, Wenger NS, Shapiro MF. The contributions of authors to multiauthored biomedical research papers. *JAMA* 1994;**271**:438–42.
10 Eastwood S, Derish P, Leash E, Ordway S. Ethical issues in biomedical research: perceptions and practices of postdoctoral research fellows responding to a survey. *Sci Eng Ethics* 1996;**2**:89–114.
11 Lock S. Lessons from the Pearce affair: handling scientific fraud. *BMJ* 1995;**310**:1547–8.
12 Marshall E. Fraud strikes top genome lab. *Science* 1996;**274**:908–10.
13 Greenfield B, Kaufman JL, Hueston WJ, Mainous AG, De Bakey L, DeBakey S. Authors vs contributors: accuracy, accountability, and responsibility. *JAMA* 1998;**279**:356–7.
14 Editorial. Games people play with authors' names. *Nature* 1997;**387**:831.
15 Horton R. The unmasked carnival of science. *Lancet* 1998;**351**:688–9.

17: Style: what it is and why it matters

MARGARET COOTER

Good organisation of the contents is the first step towards producing a "stylish" paper, and the preceding chapters have dealt with gathering the information you need and structuring your article. The next step is good writing – good scientific style. A further step, house style, will be added by the journal's editorial staff.

A scientific article needs to be fit for its purpose – the communication of information. When drafting or revising your paper, you need to keep three main things in mind: be clear, be accurate, and be concise.

Clarity

Authors of scientific papers are so familiar with their subject that they risk being unclear to their readers. Each specialty has its buzzwords and jargon, but the language of medical conversation often isn't appropriate for clear communication with readers from outside the specialty or for readers whose first language isn't English.

By paying attention to grammar and punctuation, and by choosing words carefully, you will communicate more clearly.

- Give readers the information they need in a convenient order and in manageable chunks.
- Define terms, such as abbreviations, that may be unfamiliar to readers.
- Use the right word – if you doubt it for an instant, check the word's meaning in a dictionary. Beware of easily confused words, like mitigate and militate.

- Use sentences with simple clear structures; these are likely to be short sentences.
- Jargon should be reserved for specialist contexts; in general writing, avoiding jargon will help you express ideas simply and directly.
- Noun clusters can be confusing – "spell them out" by adding appropriate prepositions: child abuse allegations = allegations of child abuse; speed reduction measures = measures to reduce speed; obstetric complication frequency = frequency of obstetric complications.
- Use the active rather than the passive voice. Say who did what: We compared the treatment group with the control group (not: The treatment and control groups were compared). Although traditional teaching is to use the passive voice in scientific articles, readers prefer active sentences, and so do many journals.
- Try not to start sentences with "there is" or "there are" – this is a deadening phrase. Usually, changing the verb will let you get rid of "there is" – and make the sentence active. "There is a report on the two programmes" is less dull when changed to "A report on the two programmes is available."
- Make sure the verbs are in the right tense and agree with the noun they refer to:

  Strengthening the capacities to deal with these problems in developing countries is important [is, not are: the verb refers to "strengthening", not "capacities" or "countries"].

- When you use this, these, they, he, she, or it, be sure that exactly what, or who, these words refer to is clear:

  If the baby does not thrive on raw milk, boil it.

- Make comparisons clear – don't assume that readers will know which two (or more) things are being compared. This is important when there are several possibilities – for example, is the comparison with another subgroup or is it with the whole population? In some cases, the comparison is dichotomous, and the comparator need not be stated:

  More women [than men] were alive five years after diagnosis.

- Know the difference between defining clauses (no comma) and commenting clauses (commas needed):

  Medical staff who often work overtime are likely to suffer from stress.
  Medical staff, who often work overtime, are likely to suffer from stress.

  Careful punctuation avoids ambiguity.

Accuracy

When furthering the body of knowledge, you don't want mistakes in your paper, or to give scope for misunderstandings.

- Use scientific conventions (SI units, symbols, Greek letters) correctly.
- Give numbers as well as percentages in results – and check your arithmetic.
- Use, but don't rely on, a spell checker – it won't tell you that a "not" is missing from your sentence.
- Check that names are spelt correctly.
- Check that reference numbers (if you are using the Vancouver system) refer to the correct reference in the reference list, and that they are in sequence in the text.
- Check that all tables and figures are referred to in the text, and that the same terms are used within the figure as are used in the figure legend.

Conciseness

Simply by being clear and accurate, you are well on the way to saying what you have to say in the briefest way possible.

- Good structure and organisation will keep the paper "tight."
- Use the simple word rather than the irritating pomposity: before (not prior to); more than (not in excess of); depends on (not is dependent upon); also (not additionally); too (not overly); indicates (not is indicative of).

- Avoid phrases like "it is well known that."
- Avoid clichés – are they actually saying anything important?
- Keep an eye out for tautology – for example, a prior history.

Critical review

When you have written and rewritten, stand back from your manuscript – put it away for a few days and then re-read it critically. Better yet, ask a trusted colleague to review it and point out anything that is ambiguous or unclear.

Box 17.1 Style makes a difference

- Good style assists effective communication
- Style should aid, not hinder, comprehension
- Clear writing helps articles be accepted for publication
- Well presented papers make editors' jobs easier
- House style gives publications consistency and identity

House style

The journal to which you submit your manuscript may supply, or have available on its website, a style sheet that sets out some basic decisions the editors have made to get consistency in layout, punctuation, capitalisation, terminology, and so on throughout the journal. For example, guidance in the *BMJ*'s "Essentials of style" (http://bmj.com/advice/stylebook/basics.shtml) includes:

- Minimal hyphenation – use hyphens only for words with non-, -like, -type, and for adjectival phrases that include a preposition (one-off event, run-in trial). Not using hyphens will help you to avoid noun clusters.
- Minimal capitalisation. Use capitals only for names and proper nouns. Don't capitalise names of studies.
- Quotation marks – please use double, not single, inverted commas for reported speech. Full stops and commas go inside quotation marks.

- Sex: avoid "he" as a general pronoun. Make the nouns (and pronouns) plural, then use "they"; if that's not possible, use "he or she"
- English, not American spelling: aetiology, oestradiol, anaemia, haemorrhage, practice (noun), practise (verb). Foetus and fetus are both acceptable in English: the *BMJ* uses fetus.
- Drugs should be referred to by their approved non-proprietary names, and the source of any new or experimental preparations should be given.

The style book used by the *BMJ*'s technical editors elaborates on these, and similar, points. It also contains a plethora of specific decisions that have had to be made – and revised – over many decades: antimalaria drugs or antimalarial drugs? capitalise job titles, or not – the Director General or the director general? when are abbreviations allowed? beta-carotene or β carotene? Moslem or Muslim, Myanmar or Burma?

Some of the principles of house style are standards of good writing; others are admittedly arbitrary, but these provide consistency throughout the publication and help to give a journal its identity.

Your proofs

Even the best writers will find changes on their proofs. This is because the journal's editorial staff will have gone through the paper to deal with possible ambiguity and to implement house style.

Technical editors (also known as copy editors or subeditors) serve as the reader's advocate, focusing on areas that a reader would find unclear or redundant. Through their exacting scrutiny of papers before publication, technical editors aim to remove the obstacles that would hinder a reader's easy grasp of the message and details of the paper, while not distorting what the author has to say.

Towards this goal they ensure that:

- the paper is free of errors of spelling and grammar (unclear antecedents, misplaced modifiers, and subject–verb agreement problems account for 80% or more of these)

- structure is clear – this may require rewording, reorganisation, adding headings, or writing transitions
- sentences that are unclear and unsupported conclusions or gaps in logic are pointed out to the author on the proof or discussed before proof stage
- jargon is eliminated or explained, so that readers unfamiliar with the field will grasp the meaning
- verbosity is eliminated
- proper names are spelt consistently
- acronyms and abbreviations are defined or spelt out on first use and used in accordance with house style throughout the paper
- arithmetic (totals in columns of tables; numbers and percentages) is correct.

Technical editors will also "tag" the paper for electronic production, and your proof may look different from the final, published format because of this.

Smooth your paper's path to publication

Make the editor's job easier – and speed your paper on its way to publication – by learning what you can about the journal's style requirements. Be sure to look at the journal's guidelines for authors or its advice to contributors, and include all the elements that are specified in the guidelines.

- Check the journal's style sheet, if there is one – it may be sent to you when your paper is accepted subject to revision, it may be published in the journal at intervals, or detailed guidance may be available on the journal's website.
- Make sure your "title page" contains all the elements published in the journal – addresses, affiliations, job titles, corresponding author, and keywords.
- Return all the necessary forms with your revised article (for example, copyright assignment, competing interests, and permissions); the editor will need to have these so that statements of funding or competing interests can be added to the article.

- Respond fully to the editor's queries on the proof. Changes have been made because something was unclear, so don't just reinstate your original wording.
- Editors are only human and do make mistakes – if the editor's changes distort your meaning, do point this out.

Further reading

Guides to writing

Albert T, ed. *The A–Z of medical writing.* London: BMJ Books, 2000.

Carey JV. *Mind the stop: a brief guide to punctuation.* London: Penguin, 1976.

Fowler H, Winchester S. *Fowler's modern English usage.* Oxford: Oxford University Press, 2002.

Goodman NW, Edwards ME. *Medical writing: a prescription for clarity.* 2nd ed. Cambridge: Cambridge University Press, 1997.

Greenbaum S, Whitcut J. *Longman guide to English usage.* London: Penguin, 1996.

Kirkman J. *Good style: writing for science and technology.* London: E&FN Spon, 1992.

O'Connor M. *Writing successfully in science.* London: Chapman & Hall, 1999.

Strunk W Jr, White EB. *The elements of style.* Boston: Allyn & Bacon, 1999.

Style manuals

American Medical Association. *Manual of style: a guide for authors and editors.* 9th ed. Philadelphia: Lippincott Williams & Wilkins, 1998.

BMJ house style. http://bmj.com/advice/stylebook/start.shtml

Council of Biology Editors. *Scientific style and format.* 6th ed. New York: Cambridge University Press, 1994.

18: Ethics of publication

MICHAEL JG FARTHING

Introduction

Ethical considerations have taken centre stage in the protection of the rights of patients and healthy volunteers in clinical research and in considering the welfare of animals used in biomedical research. As a consequence, healthcare law and ethics has found a clearly defined position in most undergraduate medical curricula. Ethical issues that relate to research integrity and the publication of research findings have lagged behind, despite the apparent increase in the number of detected causes of serious research misconduct in North America, Europe, and elsewhere.

As editor of a specialist journal, I saw many examples of research and publication misconduct, including redundant publication (an attempt to publish data that had already been published in another journal), "salami slicing" (publishing a study piecemeal, when a single, high quality paper would have been preferable), papers submitted without the knowledge or consent of co-authors, and overt fraud in the forms of plagiarism and fabrication.[1,2] Unlike some countries in the world, the United Kingdom has no regulatory agency that deals with research misconduct, although serious cases involving medical practitioners may be reported to the General Medical Council (GMC).

Concern is that research misconduct has become more frequent during the past two decades. It is difficult to be certain whether this perceived increase is a true increase in the number of misdemeanours *committed*, but there is no doubt that the number of serious cases of research misconduct that have been *detected* has increased during this period. Stephen Lock, a past editor of the *BMJ*, has documented known or suspected cases of research misconduct in the United Kingdom, the United States, Australia, Canada, and other countries.[3] In the United Kingdom, many cases involve fabrication of clinical trial data, most commonly by general practitioners – although hospital clinicians have been guilty of similar offences. Fraud in laboratory experimentation appears less common, although in a number of notorious cases in the United States and United Kingdom, the results of laboratory experiments have been fabricated, falsified, or misrepresented.[3]

Research misconduct in the modern era is often considered to have started with William Summerlin, an immunologist at the Sloan–Kettering Institute in New York, who in 1974 used a black felt tip pen to colour patches of transplanted skin in white mice! More recently in 1997 in Germany, research leaders Herrman and Brach were investigated for serious research fraud and were found to have fabricated data in 47 publications. In one case, they used the same autoradiograph image in different orientations to represent different time points in the "same experiment". Research misconduct is not limited to biomedicine, as exemplified by the extraordinary series of fabrications in the field of nanotechnology published in *Nature* and *Science*. Reports of major plagiarism continue to be detected, as does misrepresentation of personal credentials in curriculum vitae.

What is publication ethics?

It is vital that scientists engaged in biomedical research should be fully informed of the ethical framework in which they should be operating. The Committee on Publication Ethics (COPE) published guidelines on *Good Publication Practice* in 1999[4] and continues to update these on a regular basis (http://www.publicationethics.org.uk). These guidelines cover a range of issues outlined in Box 18.1.

Study design and ethical approval

Study design

A poorly designed study unable to answer the research question posed should be regarded as unethical. The design of the study– including patient numbers, controls, experimental methods, and data analysis, etc. – should all be clearly articulated

> **Box 18.1 Key issues in publication ethics**
> - Data analysis and presentation
> - Authorship
> - Conflicts of interest
> - Peer review
> - Redundant publication
> - Plagiarism
> - Duties of editors
> - Media relations
> - Advertising
> - Research misconduct

in a written protocol. In clinical studies, power calculations should be performed to ensure that the number of subjects to be included in the study will be large enough to give a definitive result. Failure to do this can be regarded as unethical. If doubt exists about the power of a study, take specialised advice; it is usually too late to do this as part of a rescue procedure at the end of the study. Local research ethics committees may withhold ethical approval until shortcomings in study design have been rectified. The final protocol should be agreed by all investigators and their contributions clearly defined.[5] It is much safer to agree the authorship of any papers that might emerge from the study at this early stage to avoid later disputes.

Ethical approval

Approval from an appropriately constituted research ethics committee is mandatory for all studies involving people, medical records, and anonymised human tissues. When study participants are unable to give fully informed consent, the research protocol should adhere closely to international guidelines, such as those of the Council for International Organisations of Medical Sciences (CIOMS). In recent years, the ethical standards for the use of human tissues in biomedical research have increased. If human tissues or body fluids have been collected for one project for which ethical approval and consent was obtained, it cannot be assumed that these archived samples can be used again without further consent. Many countries now attempt to minimise the number of animals used in biomedical research. It should be assumed that no journal will publish human or animal studies that do not conform to the ethical standards of the country in which the journal is published.

Regular reviews of research findings should be made, including examination of the original research records. Any protocol changes during the course of the study should be agreed by all investigators. Original research records should be retained for 15 years by the institution in which the work was carried out.

Data analysis

The approach to data analysis should be clearly stated in the protocol; deviations such as *post hoc* analyses and/or data exclusion should be agreed by all investigators and disclosed in the paper. The potential now to electronically manipulate data – particularly images such as immunoblots, gels, audioradiographs, histology, and immunohistochemistry – is enormous. Original images should always be retained, and any manipulation procedures should be disclosed.

Authorship

The International Committee of Medical Editors (the Vancouver Group) has produced guidelines on authorship that demand that each author must have contributed substantially throughout the process (Box 18.2).[6] In the past "gift" (or "honorary") authorship has been employed widely. It is felt, however, that this is no longer acceptable and that the concept that the professor or head of department should inevitably find his or her way on to a paper simply because the work was performed in the department is not enough to warrant authorship. Each contributor should be able to state clearly at the end of the paper how they participated in the study. Each author must take public responsibility for the work published in the paper, although, with the multidisciplinary nature of much of the work that is performed currently, it is usually advisable to have one individual, usually the senior investigator, to act as *guarantor.*

The three conditions of authorship must all be met. Participation solely in the acquisition of funding or the collection of data does not justify authorship. General supervision of the research group also is insufficient for authorship.

Box 18.2 Authorship (from reference[6])

Authorship credit should be based only on substantial contributions to:

- Conception and design or analysis and interpretation of data; *and*
- drafts of the article or critical revisions for important intellectual content; *and*
- final approval of the version to be published.

Conflicts of interest

Conflicts of interest, or competing interests, are probably more common than most of us like to admit. Competing interests can involve all participants in the publication process, including authors, reviewers, editors, and indeed the journal owners or publishers. A competing interest might be something that when revealed at some point after publication means that a reasonable reader might feel misled or deceived. The existence of competing interests is not a crime as long as they are disclosed. Reviewers also have competing interests; he or she may be a direct competitor, for example, and may wish to retard the publication of work. The journal owner or publisher may attempt to persuade editors to publish material that may be advantageous to the journal financially, at the expense of compromising scientific or academic standards. If in doubt, disclose. It has been often quoted that disclosure is almost a panacea.

Peer review

Peer review is the process used to assess the value of papers submitted to a journal with the ultimate aim of improving the quality of the paper. The conventional approach to peer review is that the authors are usually unaware of the identity of the reviewers, whereas the reviewers do know the identity of the authors. It is argued that this enables the reviewer to give a frank opinion of the work without fear of retribution. It has been considered, however, that this is an intrinsically unfair approach and, although it protects the reviewer, it may expose the author to unfair attack, particularly if the reviewer has competing scientific or other academic interests.[7] "Open" peer review has been proposed to enhance the quality of the review, although this outcome has been hard to prove by formal evaluation. Concerns exist however that younger reviewers may be excessively exposed, particularly when commenting on the imperfections of a paper from one of the "giants" in the field. The relationship between the author, the editor, and the peer reviewer is a confidential interaction. The manuscript should only be passed on to a colleague or other individual with the editor's permission. A reviewer or editor should not use information contained in such a paper for his or her own benefit.

Redundant publication

Redundant publication (sometimes referred to as duplicate or triplicate publication) is the term used when two or more papers that overlap in a major way are published in different journals without cross-reference.[8] If the same paper is published on two or more occasions, then the biomedical literature can become biased towards a particular hypothesis or treatment modality. This is particularly hazardous with respect to clinical trials involving a new drug and the potential that this can have on biasing subsequent meta-analyses.

In some situations, however, it is entirely reasonable to republish already published material. Publication of an abstract as part of the proceedings of a scientific meeting does not constitute redundant publication, but full disclosure should be made when the full paper is submitted. Previous publication of a paper in another language is also acceptable, as long as it is disclosed. It is not uncommon for two or more papers involving the same or similar patient database to be published in sequence. Authors should disclose this to the editor and make cross-reference to previous papers.

Plagiarism

Plagiarism is the use of another individual's published work or unpublished ideas without attribution. Both scientific papers and grant proposals have been used as targets for plagiarism within the field of biomedicine. The growing reservoir of electronic material and its ease of accessibility have probably facilitated the use of plagiarism to enhance authors' apparent productivity. Plagiarism may be used in some instances as a device to cover up language difficulties for those for whom English is not the first language. Authors should always be encouraged to seek help in preparing their manuscript if language is a problem and not resort to using the words of others.

Duties of editors

Editors are the custodians of the biomedical literature and have the responsibility for maintaining high standards in research and publication ethics. The editor, however, must balance the interests of the many stakeholders in the journal, including readers, authors, editorial staff including associate editors, editorial board members, the owner and/or publisher, advertisers, and the media. Competing interests may exist between stakeholders, and the editor's duty is to ensure that these do not damage the stakeholders or the journal. Editors should have in place a transparent process by which decisions are made to accept or reject a paper for publication. They should not be reluctant to publish work that challenges previously published studies in their journal, and they should not reject studies with negative results. Editors must be willing to act promptly if subsequently it becomes apparent that a published paper has been published previously or contains fraudulent data. Editors should place a notice in the journal to indicate redundant publication or should formally retract the article after previously informing the authors of their intention. Retraction does not correct the paper records, however, such that retracted papers may continue to be cited without reference to their dubious content.[9]

Media relations

Major medical breakthroughs now attract considerable media attention. Journalists frequently attend medical meetings where they will encounter unpublished research. It is now quite common for major discoveries to be reported in a newspaper before they appear in peer reviewed journals. Authors should be encouraged to arrange for their work to be published simultaneously in the biomedical literature and the mass media. Authors should give a balanced account of their work, drawing attention to both the strengths and weaknesses of the study. Analysis of a series of press releases has indicated

---

Box 18.3 Research misconduct

Errors of judgement

- Inadequate study design
- Bias
- Self delusion
- Inappropriate statistical analysis

Misdemeanours ("trimming and cooking")

- Data manipulation
- Data exclusion
- Suppression of inconvenient facts

Fraud

- Fabrication
- Falsification
- Plagiarism

---

that the information provided to journalists plays excessively on the strengths of the studies reported and as such tends to be unbalanced.

Research misconduct

Research misconduct represents a spectrum ranging from errors of judgement (mistakes made in good faith) through what have been regarded as minor misdemeanours, so called "trimming and cooking" to blatant fraud, usually categorised as fabrication, falsification, and plagiarism (Box 18.3).

All stakeholders in the publishing process have the responsibility to be vigilant for possible breaches of research and publication ethics, and they should be willing to act as a "whistleblower." Informal surveys suggest that many investigators have suspected colleagues of research misconduct.[3,10] People are reticent about making accusations against a colleague because of the inevitable personal difficulties that might result – irrespective of whether the accusations are eventually found to be true. Information derived through this route, however, is probably the most important for exposing scientific dishonesty – it being relatively difficult to detect reliably research and publication misconduct through the peer review process. "Whistleblowers" are usually protected by anonymity in the early stages of an investigation and, in the United Kingdom, the Public Interest

Disclosure Act 1998 has provided additional legal protection for all "whistleblowers" in the workplace. This added protection has the disadvantage that it might encourage a malcontent colleague to make false allegations behind the screen of anonymity. Experience in the United States, however, would indicate that most complaints are bona fide.

A number of published guidelines describe how institutions should investigate possible research misconduct. The Royal College of Physicians, London, has indicated that every institution should have its own system to manage complaints of scientific misconduct and has suggested a procedure as to how to take the process forward.[11] Similar guidance has been provided by the United Kingdom's Medical Research Council.[12] Other countries, such as the United States, Norway, Denmark, and other European countries, have established national agencies to deal with research integrity.[13] Currently in the United Kingdom, the GMC is responsible for considering cases for research misconduct amongst clinical investigators. Interest is increasing, however, in setting up an independent advisory group within the United Kingdom to monitor the handling of research misconduct cases and to advise on their investigation.[14-16]

Prevention of research and publication misconduct

The widespread nature of research and publication misconduct in all its forms and degrees of severity indicates that existing control measures are inadequate. Improved methods for the detection of misconduct are required, as is the increased vigilance of research supervisors, laboratory co-workers, and all those involved in the publication process. Even if "policing" of research were made more effective, it would not address the fundamental issue of why some individuals advertently or inadvertently betray their responsibilities as a scientist or clinical investigator. Clear guidance on ethics should be emphasised during research training and in all institutions actively involved in research.[17] This should be accompanied, however, by endorsement of the research ethos of quality rather than quantity. A variety of other interventions may also assist (Box 18.4).

The key step in the prevention of research and publication misconduct is education. Institutional guidelines should be available to all researchers as they join a new institution, and

Box 18.4 Prevention of research and publication misconduct

Education

- Research training
- Research ethics
- Publication ethics

The research

- Protocol driven
- Establish contributors and collaborators

  - Define roles
  - Agree protocol
  - Agree presentation of results

- Define methodology for data analysis

  - Statistical advice

- Ethical approval
- Project and personal licence (Home Office)
- Supervision

  - Identify *guarantor*
  - Good communication
  - Ensure *good clinical practice*
  - Meticulous record keeping

The publication

- Disclose conflict of interest
- Disclose previous publications
- Approval by *all* contributors
- Submit to one journal at a time
- Assume research data audit

formal instruction in research and publication ethics should be part of research training and a component of all taught and non-taught courses.

Close supervision of a research project is an essential component of research integrity. Research misconduct may be more prevalent when investigators are isolated, possibly believing that "they can get away with it because no one else will know." Inadequate review of raw data by a project supervisor may facilitate falsification or fabrication in large prestigious departments in which young investigators feel excessive pressure to produce results. Research integrity is dependent on good communication between contributors, with frequent discussion on the progress of the project and openness about any difficulties encountered in adhering to the research protocol. Protocol changes should be agreed by all. *Good clinical practice* guidelines should be adhered to in all clinical studies. Record keeping must be of the highest quality. By law, case report forms from all clinical trials and other clinical studies must be kept for 15 years. Laboratory investigators must keep records of all experiments performed, which include original data printouts and any other paper or photographic record of experimental results. These should be attached to the appropriate page in a laboratory notebook. Laboratory research records should be retained in the department in which the work has been performed and should be available for review for at least 15 years.

References

1 Farthing MJG. Research misconduct. *Gut* 1997;**41**:1–2.
2 Farthing MJG. Retractions in *Gut* 10 years after publication. *Gut* 2001;**48**:285–6.
3 Lock S. Research misconduct 1974–1990: an imperfect history. In: Lock S, Wells F, Farthing M, eds. *Fraud and misconduct in biomedical research*. 3rd ed. London: BMJ Publishing Group, 2001:51–63.
4 White C, eds. *The COPE Report 1999. Annual Report of the Committee on Publication Ethics*. London: BMJ Books, 1999.
5 Smith R. Authorship: time for a paradigm shift? *BMJ* 1997;**314**:992.
6 International Committee of Medical Journal Editors. Uniform requirements for manuscripts submitted to biomedical journals. *Ann Intern Med* 1997;**126**:36–47.
7 Smith R. Peer review: reform or revolution? Time to open up the black box of peer review. *BMJ* 1997;**315**:759–60.
8 Doherty M. The misconduct of redundant publication. *Ann Rheum Dis* 1996;**55**:83–5.
9 Budd JM, Sievert ME, Schultz TR. Phenomena of retraction. *JAMA* 1998;**280**:296–7.
10 Wilmshurst P. The code of silence. *Lancet* 1997;**349**:567–9.
11 Working Party. *Fraud and misconduct in medical research. Causes, investigation and prevention*. London: Royal College of Physicians, 1991.
12 Medical Research Council. *Policy and procedure for inquiring into allegations of scientific misconduct*. Mitcham: Aldridge Print Group, 1997.
13 Nylenna M, Andersen D, Dahlquist G, Sarvas M, Aakvaag A. Handling of scientific dishonesty in the Nordic countries. *Lancet* 1999;**354**:57–61
14 Smith R. Misconduct in research: editors respond. *BMJ* 1997;**315**:201–2.
15 Farthing MJG. An editor's response to fraudsters. *BMJ* 1998;**316**:1729–31.
16 Farthing M, Horton R, Smith R. UK's failure to act on research misconduct. *Lancet* 2000;**356**:2030.
17 Medical Research Council. *Good research practice*. London: MRC, 2000.

19: Electronic publishing

CRAIG BINGHAM

Once upon a time

When I first began working for a medical journal in 1990, articles were always submitted on paper. The review process was carried out by mail, although the practice of faxing a copy of the paper to reviewers was becoming more common. The editing of accepted manuscripts was done by marking up the paper copy with red and blue pen. A copy of this marked up manuscript would be sent to the author for approval, and any author's changes would be transferred manually to the editorial copy. Marked up papers were then sent to typesetters, who retyped the entire manuscript to produce galley proofs – long strips of shiny white paper that we would read and mark for correction before sending them back to the typesetter. When corrected galleys were finalised, these were handed to the layout designer, who worked with a razor and glue to cut and paste galleys into pages. These pages were then sent to the filmmaker to be photographed, and from the resulting films, page proofs and ultimately printer's plates would be produced. The journal was printed, and no electronic version existed. The internet existed, but nobody outside some specialised academic communities had heard of it, and there was no world wide web (although it was later in 1990, in October, that Tim Berners-Lee first invented the term).[1]

Twelve years later, at the same medical journal, articles are usually submitted via email, accompanied by an electronic submission form that the authors have retrieved from our website. The review process is usually conducted via email. Accepted manuscripts are edited and style tagged in Word, which is the word processing program used by most authors, and the edited copy is emailed to the author, who makes author's corrections in the file. The manuscript editors use Word's "track changes" feature to check what the author has done before they electronically transfer the file to the production department. There, the Word file is imported into the page layout program, where style tags are converted into standard generalised mark up language (sgml). A large part of the page layout is automatic, and when the details have been completed and the proofs checked, the electronic file is transferred to the printer in portable document format (pdf). Colour proofs and printer's plates are generated directly from the pdf files. Meanwhile, the internet version of the journal, in both hypertext mark up language (html) and pdf, is generated from the same sgml files used to produce the print version.

In short, 12 years has seen a thorough transformation of the communication systems and production processes used by the journal for which I work. A similar transformation has affected most scientific journals. Some have gone even further (see Chapter 8 for a description of journals that use web based manuscript submission and peer review), and new journals exist entirely in the publication space created by the internet.

Electronic publishing – choices and links

Electronic communications are transforming journals, and this is creating new opportunities and choices for authors.

As long as an internet link is available in your home or workplace, it is easier and cheaper than ever before to submit articles to journals – wherever they might be. From the journals' perspective, the internet means it is possible to reach new readers around the world more easily and cheaply than ever before. Although many journals maintain a national or regional focus, many others are seeking to internationalise their content and cater to a world audience. This means that everyone has more places to publish, and these places have become easier to find.

Authors can now use PubMed (http://www.ncbi.nlm.nih.gov/entrez/query.fcgi) to search for articles in their subject area, identify journals that carry that subject, review abstracts to assess the standard of work published, search out the journal's internet site (this is often as simple as clicking on a link in PubMed to be taken directly to the journal's site), read the guidelines for submissions, and zap off a submission by the appropriate channel.

Factors that might influence your choice of journal

I shall not discuss factors such as the specialisation of the journal or its prestige value, as indicated by its "impact factor" or some other measure, but electronic publishing has introduced some new considerations that deserve to be highlighted:

Speed of publication

Anecdotal evidence from journals that conduct their manuscript submission and peer review processes via the internet are that these are faster than the paper based alternatives. It is not just a matter of electronic communication being faster than post (although that in itself can save weeks in relation to an international submission); there also seems to be an immediacy about electronic communications that encourages editors, reviewers, and authors to respond more promptly. This may be something of a novelty effect that will wear off, but it may also represent the greater efficiency of electronic document systems compared with paper systems. If so, the extent to which it is true will depend partly on how "user friendly" the journal's system is, and this varies from journal to journal.

Some journals are now offering "fast track" publication to authors whose articles have special importance or immediate implications for clinical care. Fast track publication can be achieved by instituting rapid review and/or by publishing the article online as soon as it is ready – ahead of the print edition. Journals with fast track procedures are highly selective about which articles are eligible for consideration, and special submission instructions are available for authors who wish to be considered.

Submission and peer review process

Many journals are adopting internet based manuscript submission and peer review. Some of these systems provide immediate confirmation of receipt of submission and web based manuscript tracking that is accessible by the author. In addition, some journals are experimenting with new, more open, peer review procedures. BioMedNet journals publish the peer review reports on accepted articles. The *BMJ* and *Medical*

Journal of Australia (*MJA*) are experimenting with peer review processes that are conducted as a more open dialogue between the authors, the reviewers, and the editors.

New publication formats

Some journals are now publishing both long and short versions of articles. Some publish articles as html and pdf files and some in formats suitable for use on personal digital assistants (palmtop computers).

Accessibility

Some journals belong to journal networks such as HighWire (http://www.highwire.org) or ScienceDirect (http://www.sciencedirect.com/), and these may increase the readership of your article by making it part of a larger database. When readers search one journal, they are led also to articles in other journals of the journal network.

Even more important, some journals make the full text of their journal available free on the internet. If they do this and they participate in PubMed's LinkOut program, any reader who finds the article on PubMed can click through to the full text. A few journals give access free from the day of publication (for example, *BMJ*, *MJA*, and *CMAJ*); others make their archives freely available a few months after publication (for example, *Proceedings of the National Academy of Sciences*). For authors who are keen to maximise the accessibility of their work, the journal's access policy is a matter to be considered.

Electronic manuscript preparation

In the new scheme of things, authors would do well to consider that they are no longer producing "papers." For most journals now, the important copy of the author's work is the electronic copy, because that is the copy that will be transformed into both electronic and printed publications. Authors can assist the efficiency of this process by taking some simple steps with their word processing documents and image files. In general, electronic documents that will work well for a publisher are simple to format and produce.

The dominance of Microsoft means that a *de facto* standard for electronic documents is the Word format (particularly Word 97 and Word 2000, which are interchangeable in almost all respects).

For many years, the *Uniform requirements for the submission of manuscripts to biomedical journals*[2] has provided a standard acceptable to hundreds of medical journals for the formatting of manuscripts on paper; this standard has saved authors from needing to reformat their work for different journals. What is lacking is a similar standard for electronic manuscripts. This means that authors who submit work to several journals may have to observe a variety of different rules on how to format and present their work. (Note to the International Committee of Medical Journal Editors and/or the World Association of Medical Editors: How about developing a *Uniform Word template for the submission of manuscripts to medical journals*? – it would save a lot of bother.) Below, I give general advice that will be suitable for submissions to most journals, but authors should always check the instructions provided by each journal before finalising their submission. Some journals may even supply a document template designed specifically for their journal.

Tips for preparing Word documents

1 It is worth while reviewing Word's behavioural preferences, which are set up under the Tools/Options submenu. In particular, several useful items can be found under the "Save" options. Turn off the "Allow fast saves" option: fast saves sound like a good idea, but they produce bloated files that are harder to email and more likely to become corrupted, particularly if the publisher attempts to translate them out of Word. Turn on "Always create backup copy" to automatically keep the penultimate version of your manuscript (useful if your master file is lost or damaged). Turn on "Save AutoRecover info" to guard against losses during computer crashes – this is particularly important if you are one of those people who forgets to save work early and often.

2 Learn how to use the Word features under the Tools/ Autocorrect submenu. Some people turn off all autocorrection features because they are disconcerted by Word's default behaviour of adjusting capitalisation and reformatting type on the fly, but these features save a lot of time once you tune

them in to match your expectations. In particular, if you have a long word like "hypergammaglobulinaemia" that you need to type repeatedly, turn on "Replace text as you type" and add it to the replacement list. Define a short unique key sequence as the text to replace with the long word (for example, replace "hy" with "hypergammaglobulinaemia") and you can improve your typing accuracy, while lowering the number of keystrokes required.

3 Keep formatting to a minimum. I have seen authors present articles as elaborate facsimiles of the journal that they are submitting to, complete with multi-column layout, embedded pictures, and a variety of fonts – a pity, as all this formatting work will be discarded by the journal as the first step towards making the author's file useful. It also annoys editors, who much prefer manuscripts in a simple one-column layout. Only use fonts that everybody has on their computers: for example, Times New Roman for your main text font and Arial as your font for headings. Turn off type justification, automatic hyphenation, and automatic paragraph numbering. On the other hand, the use of bold, italic, superscript, and subscript text as appropriate is good.

4 Use styles and style tagging rather than formatting the article paragraph by paragraph. This makes it much easier to format an article as you write and easier again if you are asked to change the formatting later. For your level 1 headings, therefore, define a Heading1 style, with the combination of font, spacing, and alignment that you want to use, and then apply this to each heading as you create it. To change all your level 1 headings later, simply redefine the style and all will be changed without having to select and manipulate each heading.

5 Format text as one continuous flow. Use a page break (Ctrl + Enter) to start a new page (for example, after your title page) not a stream of hard returns. Some journals prefer you to put only one hard return between each paragraph, others prefer two, but more than two is a nuisance. Do not break the article up with Word's section breaks.

6 Do not use a string of spaces as a formatting device in tables or anywhere else. Although text formatted this way may look correct on your computer, it becomes distorted

once it is translated from Word into the publisher's desktop publishing system. To set text at a certain position on the page, use a tab – not a string of tabs, but one tab, defined to be in the right place (to set tabs, select "Tabs" under the "Format" menu, or view the ruler and drag the tabs to the right locations).

7   Keep table formatting simple and consistent. A common error is to place a column of separate items into a single table cell, with each item separated by a hard return: instead each data item should have a table cell of its own. Sometimes tables are formatted with tabs instead of cells: in this case, the key is to set the tab stops for the whole table so that one tab equals one column.

8   Most publishers ask you not to embed image files or other objects in your Word document. Most publishers' production systems will choke on this non-text material when they try to import your Word file, and images are frequently processed by people within the publisher's production team who will not be dealing with your text. Image files should be sent as separate files (other requirements of image files are discussed below). The same goes for Excel spreadsheets or charts. If you are embedding images in the file, it is probably best to do it at the end, after the text and references.

9   Be prepared to send the data used to generate graphs. Some publishers will use the data to regenerate the graphs according to their own style rules. In such a case, it helps if you send only the data that are actually shown in the graphs – not the spreadsheet with all of the data generated in the study.

10 Present the reference list as plain text at the end of the file, unless you are submitting to a journal that specifically endorses the use of Word's endnotes and footnotes. Word's endnotes and footnotes have some advantages in terms of automatic ordering and numbering, but they exist in a separate text flow and are easily lost or garbled during translations from Word to other formats. If you like to use endnotes to contain the reference list during the drafting stages, you can convert them to plain text by saving your file in plain text format, but you will lose all formatting (including bold and italic) at the same time.

What about pdf?

Adobe's portable document format is designed to produce a file that will be viewed and printed from any computer that has the free Adobe Acrobat reader software installed. If you have the complete Acrobat program (not just the free reader), a pdf file can be created from Word, or many other applications.

The chief advantage of a pdf is that you can be sure that the file you created can be viewed and printed exactly as you created it. This is not necessarily true of a Word file, which may be reformatted when it is displayed or printed from somebody else's computer. However, pdf files are not editable in the same way as word processor files. Some publishers will ask for, or even create, a pdf file of your manuscript for use during the peer review process, but a Word file will also be required for editing and production. Other publishers only want a Word file. Don't send a pdf if the publisher wants the manuscript sent in Word or any other word processor format.

Tips for preparing images

The most common error in preparing electronic images is to make them too small. Images appear on a computer screen at a resolution of 72 or 96 pixels per inch (ppi), but to achieve a similar quality of reproduction in print, an image will be printed at 300 dots per inch (dpi). An image that appears on screen as four inches (100 mm) wide at 72 ppi will only be one inch (25 mm) wide when printed at 300 dpi. When this image is printed at four inches wide, jagged edges will show instead of smooth curves and tone blocks instead of smooth tone transitions.

No effective way exists to increase the resolution of an image beyond its original size, and if an image is reduced in size and saved, picture data is permanently lost. Image files therefore have to be created and saved at high resolution. For a colour image that is to be printed as 4×4 inches, the required size is $(4 \times 300) \times (4 \times 300) = 1200 \times 1200 = 1\,440\,000$ dots. In many image formats (for example, tagged image file format, or tiff), each dot will take eight bits (one byte) to store, so the image file will be 1·44 megabytes – enough to fill a floppy disk and 15–30 times the size of most image files viewed over the internet.

Compression techniques can reduce the size of the image file, but again caution is required. Zip compression is safe, because it uses an algorithm that packs the data tighter without throwing any of it away. Compression during which files are saved in jpeg format, however, works by discarding picture data – the algorithm is very clever, and often quite a lot of compression can be applied without any discernible loss of picture quality. Flaws not evident when viewing the image on screen, however, may show up in a printed copy – particularly in the high quality printed copy produced by a journal's press.

Most software allows you to select the level of compression you wish to apply when saving a file in jpeg format, and it is safest to select the option for large file size (maximum picture quality).

Publishers have varying requirements for image file formats, but tiff and jpeg are usually safe choices. For vector images (that is, images such as graphs and charts generated by a computer drawing package, in which the data are described as lines and areas (vectors) rather than as single pixels), eps is the best file format to use. Whatever file format you are using, it is useful to send information about the image and how it was produced along with the electronic file.

The electronic future

Electronic publishing could be said to be the central technology of the scientific medical literature, but it is far from a mature technology. Many of the recommendations for manuscript preparation made in this chapter will date rapidly, and the core requirements of "computer literacy" are changing constantly. We are approaching a globalised medical literature, in which it will be increasingly easy to move from article to article, journal to journal, without interruption. Just exactly how this will be paid for remains uncertain. Commercial publishers tend to look for "pay-per-view" or subscription revenues – an Internet with regular tollbooths – while many academic institutions, governmental authorities, and some professional organisations favour hidden subsidy models in which internet access to the literature is apparently free to the reader. Technologies and business models for both systems are developing competitively. Readers' preferences may be decisive, but authors are also influential – through their choice of where to submit articles for publication.

References

1 W3C. *A Little History of the World Wide Web.* Available from http://www.w3.org/History.html (accessed 31 Mar 2003).
2 International Committee of Medical Journal Editors. *Uniform Requirements for Manuscripts Submitted to Biomedical Journals.* http://www.icmje.org (accessed 31 Mar 2003).

Index

Page numbers in *italic* refer to tables or boxed material